The
VIAGRA ALTERNATIVE

The
VIAGRA
ALTERNATIVE

The Complete
Guide
to Overcoming
Erectile Dysfunction
Naturally

MARC BONNARD, M.D.

Healing Arts Press
Rochester, Vermont

Healing Arts Press
One Park Street
Rochester, Vermont 05767
www.InnerTraditions.com

Healing Arts Press is a division of Inner Traditions International

Thanks to Deborah Straw, Lee Wood, and Rowan Jacobsen for their contributions to this project.

Note to the reader: This book is intended as an informational guide. The remedies, approaches, and techniques described herein are meant to supplement, and not to be a substitute for, professional medical care or treatment. They should not be used to treat a serious ailment without prior consultation with a qualified health care professional.

LIBRARY OF CONGRESS CATALOGING-IN-PUBLICATION DATA
Bonnard, Marc.
    The viagra alternative : the complete guide to overcoming erectile dysfunction naturally / Marc Bonnard.
        p.   cm.
    Includes bibliographical references and index.
    ISBN 0-89281-789-5 (alk. paper)
        1. Impotence—Alternative treatment.   I. Title.
RC889.B586   1999
616.6'9206—dc21   99-40743
                                                CIP

Printed and bound in Canada

10 9 8 7 6 5 4 3 2 1

Text design and layout by Crystal H. H. Roberts
This book was typeset in Bookman

"I will show you a philtre without potions, without herbs, without witches' incantations. It is this: If you wish to be loved, then love."

Seneca

CONTENTS

INTRODUCTION

A VIAGRA REVOLUTION?

You've seen the headlines. *New pill revolutionizes treatment of impotence.* Maybe you've even seen the numbers: more than a million prescriptions written per month shortly after the drug's release, making it the most successfully released drug in the history of medicine. So those headlines didn't lie; any drug that generates that many users and suffuses the culture so thoroughly that it creates a permanent industry of running jokes has indeed triggered some sort of revolution.

But what kind of revolution has it been? And has anything really changed?

For many men the answer is yes. Viagra is an effective medication, and in two out of three men with physical erectile problems it does indeed help to produce an erection. So if you expected to open this book and find a polemic on the evils of the drug Viagra,

1

you're in for a surprise. I believe Viagra is, overall, a good thing, and there are two main reasons why I believe so. One, as you'll see in a later chapter that examines the previous medical treatments for erectile dysfunction—which can only be called ugly—Viagra is so much easier and more pleasant to use that it has truly improved the lives of millions of men.

But the more important positive effect of the "Viagra revolution" is cultural, not medical. Viagra has managed to do what countless doctors and psychologists have been unable to do for decades: it has finally removed the taboo from the subject of impotence and made it an acceptable topic for discussion—in the media, in the home, and with a doctor.

The importance of this change cannot be overstated. Before Viagra, it is estimated that for every one man brave enough to actually broach the subject with his doctor, there were nine others who suffered in silence. And though this is still a problem, the situation is changing, and changing fast. In 1997, the year before Viagra's approval by the FDA, 2.8 million men in the United States visited their doctors because of erectile dysfunction. In 1998, with Viagra dominating the media and available for prescription, that number jumped to 4.8 million. I believe the number will continue to climb, though we still have a long way to go before all of the estimated 30 million men in the United States with erectile dysfunction will have sought help.

Before we go any further, we should discuss terminology. The term *impotence,* still prevalent in the media and the culture at large, is no longer used by experts on the subject because of its emotional baggage, which tends to imply loss of power and capabilities far beyond the arena of sexual functioning. *Erectile dysfunction* is the term used by experts in the field because it more clearly defines the problem, and it is the term I'll use in this book. As you know if you've seen Bob Dole's Viagra advertisements, this term is often abbreviated ED, and in the interest of efficiency I'll do likewise.

So ED is out of the closet and recognized as the devastating and widespread health condition it is. Great. And everyone with the condition should get some Viagra and their problems will be solved, right?

Wrong. For while Viagra is an acceptable and fairly effective way to treat ED, it is rarely the *best* way. Erectile dysfunction is not natural. If you have ED, something is wrong. Something needs fixing, and Viagra does not fix the problem, it just enables you to keep doing what it is you want to do (have sex), while the problem slowly gets worse—to the point where the drug may not work anymore. If your muffler breaks on your car and the racket is so loud that you can't comfortably ride in it any longer, you don't simply turn up the radio and keep driving; you go to a mechanic and get the car fixed. Much more so than your broken muffler, erectile dysfunction is like the dead canary in a coal mine—a warning sign that there is a deeper systemic problem that needs addressing. Erectile dysfunction can be the first sign of clogged arteries, hypertension, diabetes, and other problems. And while a responsible doctor will examine all patients with ED for these other diseases, too many do not. This problem is also greatly compounded by the phenomenon of Viagra being in such demand that it is routinely prescribed over the Internet by doctors who never set eyes on the patients they are "treating." A thriving Viagra black market has also sprung up, with men ordering the drug from Mexico (where it is sold over-the-counter) or from other Internet sources, entirely circumventing a physician's approval and allowing life-threatening conditions to go unnoticed.

A second troubling effect of the Viagra revolution is much less obvious, but may ultimately be even more damaging. As is clear by the media's spin on the story and the fact that men with full sexual function were eager to purchase Viagra on the black market, erections have practically become synonymous with good sex. Many jokes about Viagra leave the unmistakable impression that simply popping a Viagra can do wonders for the sex life of perfectly healthy couples! Viagra has even become popular on the club scene, sold for $20 a pill and taken with the drug Ecstasy in a combination called "Sextasy"—a practice that some specialists worry could be causing permanent penile damage. The truth of the matter is that most mature people find that sex without affection and intimacy gets old pretty fast—no matter how hard the erection. And a pill that creates a limited window of time when an erection can occur tends to force the issue in ways not always in sync with the natural feelings of tenderness, love, and arousal of the man's partner, leading to emotional strain and conflict. Sex is meant to be the ultimate consummation of powerful feelings between two people, and that can easily be lost by the wayside when all the focus is on an erection.

That's where this book comes in. It is for the millions of men—and women—who, for a number of reasons, know that Viagra is not the answer for them. If you want to know about alternatives that work on the health of the whole body and allow you to naturally attain an erection whenever you want, then this book is for you. If you have ED, suspect that it stems, at least partially, from relationship problems, and want to work on those problems with a sex therapist instead of simply taking Viagra and letting the relationship deteriorate, then this is the book for you, too.

This book is for many others as well. If your ED is physical and you are wise enough to want to address the root causes of the problem by focusing on dietary and lifestyle changes that can not only restore erectile function but also make you feel better and live longer, you'll find help inside.

Even if you don't have ED, this book may be for you. People have been making love a lot longer than doctors have been prescribing Viagra, and many of them have turned it into an art. So in this book I include information on helpful sexual techniques, along with information on vitamin supplements, exercises, and mood-enhancing tips that can improve anyone's sex life.

And we haven't even gotten to the herbal alternatives yet. Many of you bought this book because it features the most complete information available on natural cures for erectile dysfunction, and I've waited until the end of the introduction to discuss it. But don't worry, I've saved the best for last. For there is an amazing range of natural substances—some new, some very old—that have been proven successful in treating sexual dysfunction. So if Viagra didn't help you, this book is definitely for you. Even if it did, but you worry about the side effects or have one of the conditions that rules out Viagra, then you'll want to know about the herbal alternatives listed here. If you simply prefer to keep pharmaceuticals out of your body and trust nature's remedies instead, this is where you'll find them. Some of these herbal alternatives are fairly new discoveries, and some have been popular in other countries, such as China, for years, but remained unknown in the United States until demand for Viagra spilled over into demand for Viagra alternatives.

The upshot of all this is that if you have erectile dysfunction, the chances of finding an effective remedy have never been so good. However, it is important that you become aware of all the choices available, and not just the ones the media considers newsworthy at any particular moment.

It is also vitally important that we keep sex in its proper context. The West has become ever more sex crazy in recent years, and we are all barraged by images of sexuality in magazines, in movies and television, and on the Internet. More often than not, the goal of these images is to sell you something. And while there is nothing wrong with sexual images, the effect of this constant bombardment is to make us all involuntary initiates into the Cult of Youth, where aging and the difficulties that are associated with it are considered unnatural, to be avoided if at all possible.

The truth is that our sex lives change as we age. Half of American males over the age of forty will be affected by erectile dysfunction at some point in their lives. This extremely high percentage is partially because we are simply living longer, and partially because our diets and lifestyles are much less healthy than they were in the past. Whatever the reason, this number is too high, and most of these men can find natural methods for improving their condition. There is no reason why older people shouldn't have sex— sex is proven to be physically and mentally beneficial—but at the same time, we don't want seventy-year-old men thinking of themselves as twenty-five-year-olds and behaving accordingly. Having too many elderly men eager to put their newly revived physical capabilities to use could lead to increased adultery and even divorce. There is a case of a ninety-four-year-old man fathering a child, and while this is great proof that the male reproductive system is never *officially* too old to work, most would agree that we don't want to see this becoming a regular occurrence.

The point is that we should keep a holistic view of the place of sex in our lives, especially if, thanks to Viagra or the methods recommended in this book, sex has only recently come back into our lives. Sex is a tremendously powerful force that can bring about great physical pleasure, improved health, and wonderful intimacy and love. But used unwisely, it can wreck homes, destroy relationships, and spread disease. It is my hope that the remedies recommended in this book, which tend to work hand in hand with the improved overall physical and mental health of the patient, will help to bring about a greater understanding of sexuality in your own life, as well as renewed enjoyment of one of the most potentially spiritual of all activities.

1 WHAT IS VIAGRA AND IS IT SAFE?

SILDENAFIL AND A DISTURBING TRAIL OF DEATHS

In order to be able to make an informed decision on whether or not Viagra is the way you want to treat your erectile dysfunction, you need to have a full understanding of what Viagra—officially known as sildenafil—is, and of how it works. It may surprise you to learn that the medication wasn't even originally intended to treat erectile dysfunction.

In the 1980s, in Great Britain, researchers began studying the properties of a new molecule: sildenafil. It had originally been unsuccessfully tested in cardiology as a dilator of blood vessels. Sildenafil proved to be of no use to cardiac patients, and the tests were discontinued. However, much to their surprise, researchers found that many of the patients asked to continue the medication. Why? When questioned, these cardiac patients, many of whose vascular problems had caused erectile dysfunction as well, admitted that they had experienced significant improvement in their erections. This observation eventually led to European clinical tests on men with erectile dysfunction.

At the 1996 annual congress of the American Urological Association, the first results of this new medication under research for the treatment of erectile dysfunction were presented. The first results in clinical research showed sildenafil to be particularly effective in men with mild physical ED. A program of worldwide research with clinical trials was undertaken, and in 1998, under the brand name Viagra, sildenafil was made available to the general public.

VIAGRA AND THE CLINICAL TRIALS

Viagra has been studied extensively in clinical trials, at doses of 25 mg, 50 mg, and 100 mg. It has been clearly demonstrated to improve erections. Viagra was evaluated in 21 randomized double-blind, placebo-controlled trials of up to six months. In these trials, Viagra was studied in more than 3,000 patients between the ages of 19 and 87, who had had erectile dysfunction for an average of five years. More than 550 patients were treated for longer than one year. Clinical testing occured in a "real world" setting.

The efficacity of Viagra was demonstrated in all 21 studies. In clinical trials, patients receiving Viagra reported a 78 percent improvent in erections versus 20 percent for a placebo pill. (Note the high placebo percentage, indicating that a significant number of patients didn't need Viagra or any other medication to overcome their ED.)

Though manufacturer Pfizer claims that the word *Viagra* was chosen at random, and *Alond* was almost chosen as the product name, the word does seem particularly rich in connotations. "Niagara" springs to mind immediately, bringing forth visions of rushing, explosive power. Niagara Falls is also, of course, the classic destination for honeymooners, so there is a subtle implication that Viagra can revive those feelings couples had during their honeymoon. "Vigor" also comes to mind—as in young, healthy men with vigorous erections.

Viagra is not an aphrodisiac. It has no effect on sex drive or libido. Thus it cannot cause an erection in the absence of stimulus: it doesn't send the message for an erection to occur, nor does it create extra blood to make the penis that much harder. So while the drug does facilitate an erection, it does not necessarily enhance one. It won't increase pleasure beyond what is felt during normal, healthy intercourse. If a man does not have erectile dysfunction, Viagra will have no effect on his erection. Similarly, a patient who has achieved success with a 50 mg dose of Viagra will find no additional benefits from a 100 mg dose. Picture a dam where the wheels that open the floodgates have rusted shut. Viagra is simply the grease that frees those wheels up and allows the water to come pouring through. It doesn't turn the wheels of its own accord, doesn't force the floodgates open any wider than they would normally go, and doesn't generate any additional water. It simply allows the dam to function as it normally would—and for most men with ED, this is certainly enough.

CONTRAINDICATIONS

No doubt you have heard the reports of hundreds of deaths linked to Viagra. At last count 220 deaths had been associated with Viagra in some way, and by the time you read this the number will have climbed further. While investigators are still determining what role Viagra played in these deaths, one thing is overwhelmingly clear: for a large group of men with erectile dysfunction, taking Viagra could cost them their lives. Pfizer does not dispute this and warns that Viagra is absolutely contraindicated in patients taking nitrates in any form and at any time. There are 125 drugs currently on the market that contain nitrates, which are commonly used to treat hypertension—high blood pressure. They work by dilating blood vessels, thereby lowering blood pressure. Viagra potentiates this effect, causing a feeling of sickness and, more importantly, a potentially dramatic drop in blood pressure. Think of a hose that is widened so that the water flows smoothly out of the end, but then is widened again, so much that only a trickle now comes out, and none gets to your flowers.

Here is a list of commonly used nitrates, all of which should never be mixed with Viagra, along with the brand names under which they are sold:

Erythatyl tetranitrate
   Cardilate
Isosorbide mononitrate
   Imdur
   Ismo
   Monoket tablets

Isosorbide dinitrate
  Dilatrate-SR
  Isordil
  Sorbitrate
Nitroglycerin
  Deponit
  Minitran
  Nitrek
  Nitro-Bid
  Nitrodisc
  Nitro-Dur
  Nitrogard
  Nitroglyn
  Nitrolingual Spray
  Nitral Ointment
  Nitrong
  Nitro-Par
  Nitrostat
  Nitro-Time
  Transdermal-Nitro
Pentaerythritol tetranitrate
  Pentritol
  Peritrate
Sodium nitroprusside

The same warning holds true for the "poppers" taken in clubs. Poppers are inhaled amyl nitrate, which can also cause a dramatic drop in blood pressure. In any case, if you need to rely on Viagra *and* poppers to have a satisfactory sexual experience, you probably have psychological issues that should be dealt with first.

Men with an anatomical deformity of the penis such as Peyronie's disease, with conditions known to produce priapism (such as anemia, multiple myeloma, and leukemia), or with retinal problems like macular degeneration and retinitis pigmentosa, should use caution in using Viagra. If it is used, doses should be kept at the absolute lowest level possible.

Men taking protease inhibitors to suppress their HIV infection may be at an increased risk of heart attack. At least one patient with HIV and no history of heart problems died of a heart attack after taking Viagra. Doctors are researching this drug interaction further, but for now other options are probably a better bet.

Before using Viagra, all men should consider their level of cardiovascular health, given the physical exertion involved in intercourse. So often being overweight causes the vascular problems that lead to both heart conditions and impotence in the first place. The body is an amazingly complex network of interacting systems; when something goes wrong with it, the whole body must be considered in the treatment if there is to be any permanent cure. In these cases the erectile dysfunction can even be seen as a self-regulating safety mechanism: the body taking care of itself. If the body was physically prepared for intercourse, it would be able to achieve an erection. That it can't is a clear sign that there are significant underlying problems, and some significant changes in lifestyle are called for.

This is where conventional medicine frequently misses the boat, and Viagra is a classic example. Treating the one symptom—erectile dysfunction—and ignoring the larger problems is tantamount to bypassing the body's own safety mechanism. It can lead to a far worse condition than erectile dysfunction: it can lead to death. This is one of the reasons why Viagra is not doing favors for as many men as the early press reports led us to believe. Men at risk of heart attack would be much better served by a program of exercise and dietary changes. This will lead to weight loss, reduction of arterial blockage, increased stamina, more energy, and even a better mood. Then, when the erection spontaneously returns, it can be seen not only as a sign that it is time to resume sexual intercourse, but also as a reward for all the hard work and dedication that has resulted in a new, improved you.

In addition to overweight men, older men who haven't enjoyed sexual relations in a long time should heed the same warnings. They, too, can die from placing too much demand on their hearts. Approximately 2 percent of heart attacks occur during sexual activity, and this number will probably be much higher among Viagra users who don't undergo proper cardiac examinations. Viagra, though certainly not responsible, may encourage a sexual confidence that exceeds a man's physical capacity. You pop a pill, and for the next hour or so your mind is completely focused on sex. You want your money's worth. An erection is on the way, it hasn't been easy to get one lately, and by god you're gonna have sex before it disappears, come hell, high water, or heart attack. Worse still, the older men most likely to find themselves in this situation are also the ones most likely not to have told their partners that they have taken Viagra (especially if their partners are much younger), and the medical personnel who treat the heart attack may administer an injection of drugs containing nitrates, which when combined with the Viagra increase the likelihood of death. The advice here is as old-fashioned and simple as it is sound: listen to your body. Don't make it do anything it isn't ready for.

The good news is that it is never too late to get back in shape, to reverse the aging process, and to once again engage in wonderful sexual intercourse. And rare is the case where this can't be achieved through behavioral changes, coupled, when necessary, with all-natural supplements that don't set a timetable for your erection.

OTHER ADVERSE SIDE EFFECTS OF VIAGRA

In clinical trials other adverse effects reported by patients receiving Viagra were generally similar and insignificant. Their intensity varied in proportion to the size of the dose. The following adverse effects were reported by patients:

EFFECT	VIAGRA	PLACEBO
Headache	16%	4%
Flushing (reddening of the face)	10%	1%
Dyspesia (upset stomach)	7%	2%
Nasal congestion	4%	2%
Urinary tract infection	3%	2%
Abnormal vision	3%	0%
Diarrhea	3%	1%
Dizziness	2%	1%
Rash	2%	1%

One unusual side effect encountered is slight color-blindness, in which the patient temporarily becomes unable to distinguish blue from green. This is probably due to Viagra's effect on the enzyme PDE-6, which is found in the retina of the eye and is closely related to the PDE-5 found in the penis. PDE-6 is involved in the phototransduction process that allows us to see colors. While Viagra is highly effective at inactivating PDE-5, and pretty much ignores the other phosphodiesterases, it is slightly effective at inactivating PDE-6. This generally only occurs with doses of 100 mg or more, and at that dosage affects about 11 percent of users, lasting from several minutes to a few hours. Interestingly, this phenomenon is most often decribed by patients who have light-colored eyes. Under most circumstances this is little more than an inconvenience, but there was a small plane crash in Maryland in 1998 in which it was speculated that the pilot, who was known to be taking Viagra, may have had trouble distinguishing the colors of the runway lights. The long-term effect of Viagra on the eyes remains unknown.

FORM

Viagra is supplied as blue, film-coated, rounded diamond-shaped tablets containing sildenafil citrate in doses of either 25, 50, or 100 mg. For most patients the recommended dose is 50 mg. One tablet of Viagra costs approximately $10 and can only be attained with a doctor's prescription. However, it is being sold on the black market—especially in countries in which it has not yet been approved—for many times that amount.

Viagra has a relatively short plasma half-life of approximately four to five hours, but the drug must not be taken more than once a day.

DISTURBING TRENDS

As a medication, Viagra has been a clear success. It has lived up to Pfizer's claims, and, when the instructions on how to use it are followed to the letter, it seems to cause only minor side effects (its long-term effects will not be known for years). As a social phenomenon, however, Viagra comes dragging many question marks.

Clearly too many men are dying due to Viagra. True, they ignored (or never saw) warnings about mixing Viagra with nitrates and other drugs, or they ignored their own cardiovascular condition. But ED is a powerfully emotional issue, so it may not be fair to tell these men, "Here is a medicine that will allow you to have sex again, but it may kill you." It is a bit like putting a pie in front of a three-year-old and saying, "This is for later; you can smell it, but don't eat it now." We know that temptation and desperation are regularly going to triumph over common sense in these situations.

The desire to obtain Viagra anonymously, due to the embarassment many men with ED feel, has driven an explosion of online pharmacies that may ultimately prove to be far more damaging than Viagra could ever be. The best of these "pharmacies" ask a few questions about your situation and other medications you may be taking; the worst are set up overseas, beyond the regulatory power of the United States, and for the right price will simply ship you whatever prescription medicines you want. In one case, the physician approving prescriptions for a domestic online pharmacy was found to be a retired veterinarian living in Mexico. And, though these online pharmacies have become vastly more popular due to Viagra, they also prescribe a host of other potentially dangerous drugs, including Demerol, Propecia, and Xanax.

Obviously, if many men begin obtaining Viagra without proper oversight by qualified physicians, and without essential preliminary and follow-up physical exams, the death toll will rise dramatically. This is why it would be so much better for the word to get out that ED can usually be successfully treated with completely natural physical, behavioral, and psychological methods.

THE BOTTOM LINE

A great deal of progress has been made in the pharmacological treatment of erectile dysfunction, and Viagra is the greatest leap forward that field has ever taken. You need only review the following chapter, on other medical treatments for erectile dysfunction, to understand why a simple pill that effectively facilitates erections is like a dream come true for some men. So let us give Viagra its due: it is a step forward, and for some men it is indeed the answer. But there is still a 20 to 50 percent chance of failure from treatment with Viagra, depending on the origin of the erectile difficulty. It is not a panacea, even for men not interested in addressing the underlying causes of their ED.

More importantly, good sex does not happen on its own. Yes, the penis is the focus of therapeutic attention. But the penis is connected to a body, which has a brain, and frequently that body is associated with another body—a partner. Regrettably, this is often forgotten in ED treatments. Restoring erectile function is one thing. For restoring good sex, it is essential to address personal and emotional factors in the sufferer, as well as conflicts in his relationship with his partner—all of which may be instrumental in causing or maintaining the present erectile disorder. Often sex therapy—which I'll discuss in a later chapter—can be extremely useful, with or without the use of natural or pharmaceutical "helpers." It is important not to neglect this ever-present component.

2 WHAT GOES UP MUST COME DOWN

CAUSES OF ERECTILE DYSFUNCTION

Erectile dysfunction is defined as the inability to achieve or maintain an erection that is sufficient for satisfactory sexual performance. Erectile dysfunction has nothing to do with sexual desire, orgasm, or ejaculation. It is simply a failure, for any of a number of reasons, to get enough blood into the penis and hold it there with enough rigidity to achieve mutually satisfying sexual intercourse. It is an affliction with severe emotional symptoms for men and their sexual partners.

There are a lot of fundamental misconceptions about erectile dysfunction, on the part of both patients and physicians. Almost always treatable, erectile dysfunction is not an inevitable consequence of old age. Today's treatments for erectile dysfunction—both allopathic and alternative—allow most men, regardless of age, to enjoy sex again.

Many men suffer from temporary loss of erectile capacity. This is perfectly normal and can be explained by fatigue, stress, temporary disinterest, an evening of too many drinks, or the uncertainties of a new relationship. Generally this is nothing to worry about, and everything returns to normal the following day. However, if the condition persists and interferes with normal sexual activity, erectile dysfunction may be occurring, and medical advice should be sought.

Erectile dysfunction can be divided between primary erectile dysfunction and secondary erectile dysfunction. Primary ED is the condition in which a man has never in his life sustained an erection sufficient to engage in the act of sexual intercourse. Secondary ED is when normal erections and orgasms have previously occurred, but have now ceased to do so.

Men suffering from ED should know that they are not alone. The National Institutes of Health estimates that as many as 30 million American men are affected by erectile dysfunction, but that only 5 to 10 percent of them have ever been treated for it. The majority of these individuals are over the age of sixty-five.

Medical studies show that about 10 percent of men have erectile dysfunction and the number rises with age to one in three men over the age of sixty and two of three over age seventy. The most comprehensive study ever done on ED, the Massachusetts Male Aging Study, surveyed 1,290 men in the Boston area and found that between the ages of 40 and 70 the probability of complete erectile dysfunction tripled from 5 to 15 percent, while the probability of moderate erectile dysfunction doubled from 17 to 34 percent. Within the same age range the probability of minimal erectile dysfunction remained constant at approximately 17 percent. Overall, 52 percent of the men studied had some degree of ED.

It should be noted that erectile dysfunction and sterility have nothing in common. Patients with ED can be perfectly fertile, but unable to get their sperm where it needs to go. Sterile men, on the other hand, can have normal erections, and their ability to have sex is not altered, but because of the low quantity or quality of their spermatozoa they are unable to impregnate a woman.

THE ANATOMY OF AN ERECTION

To understand what causes erectile dysfunction—what goes wrong—we first need to understand what occurs when everything goes right. An erection may seem like the simplest thing in the world: the penis gets hard. But what makes that penis hard? There is no bone in it, after all, or it would never become flaccid. Instead, "hardness" is caused by the penis filling with blood to the point where the pressure is strong enough that there is no "give" left. Think of the tire of a car: without air it is perfectly soft, but when filled the pressure makes it very hard.

Why then, you ask, isn't the penis always hard? Blood is always circulating through it, after all. To answer this we need to learn a little about the penis's anatomy.

The penis is an organ with paired erectile chambers called the *corpora cavernosa* running almost its entire length. These cylinders are surrounded and held in place by a fibrous sheath called the *tunica albug-*

MALE REPRODUCTIVE ORGANS

Bladder

Pubic bone

Prostatic gland

Corpora cavernosa

Glans (corpus spongiosum)

Foreskin

Urinary meatus

Ureter

Rectum

Seminal vesicle

Ejaculatory duct

Urethra

Vas deferens

Anus

Epididymis

Testis

Scrotum

CROSS SECTION OF PENIS

Superficial dorsal vein

Dorsal arteries

Tunica albuginea (fibrous coat)

Deep dorsal vein

Helicine arteriole

Cavernosal (erection) artery

Lacunar spaces (sinuses)

Corpus cavernosum (erectile tissue)

Corpus spongiosum

Urethra

Penile skin

inea. (To continue our tire metaphor, the corpora cavernosa would be the tube and the tunica albuginea would be the tread.) The corpora cavernosa are filled with spongy tissue rich in tiny pool-shaped blood vessels called *lacunar spaces,* which are surrounded by smooth muscles and supported by elastic fibrous tissue composed of collagen. The lacunar spaces are supplied with blood through small blood vessels called *helicine arteries*, which in turn are branches of the blood supplier for the entire penis, the penile artery. In the penis's normal flaccid state, these spaces are empty because the smooth muscle surrounding them is contracted, constricting the helicine arteries and preventing blood from flowing in.

Like all the other organs of the body, the penis does need a constant minimal supply of blood to maintain healthy tissue. This inflow of blood through the arteries is then drained away by a system of veins that runs just beneath the tunica albuginea, where it meets the spongy tissue of the corpora cavernosa.

The smooth muscle cells of the corpora cavernosa play a key role in initiating an erection. Paradoxically, they must *relax* in order for an erection to occur. By doing so, when signaled by the brain, they allow blood to flow through the helicine arteries, filling the pool-shaped lacunar spaces. The arteries also dilate to allow for the greater flow of blood. As the lacunar spaces fill, the corpora cavernosa inflate, pushing against the tunica albuginea as they do so. A neat engineering trick is that, because the veins that drain the penis are located between the tunica albuginea and the corpora cavernosa, as the corpora cavernosa swells it squeezes these veins against the less flexible tunica albuginea, pinching them off and preventing the new inflow of blood from being drained away. Penile pressure increases to approach mean arterial blood pressure and penile rigidity develops. This is an erection.

Once the smooth muscle of the penis stops receiving signals from the brain to produce an erection, it contracts again, preventing further inflow of blood to the penis. Without this blood, the pressure inside the corpora cavernosa drops just enough to allow the veins to again begin to drain blood out of the penis, further reducing pressure and allowing increasingly faster drainage to occur, and the penis quickly returns to its flaccid state.

An additional part of the penis we have thus far ignored is the *corpus spongiosum,* located in the groove beneath the two cylinders of the corpora cavernosa. Like them, this chamber is composed of spongy tissue that fills with blood during an erection, though to a lesser extent than the corpora cavernosa. More important, the corpus spongiosum contains the urethra, the tube through which urine and semen travel. Though cylindrical for most of its length, the corpus spongiosum differentiates at its end to form the glans, or head, of the penis, one of the areas of the body densest in nerve endings and thus one of the most sensitive, making it a central player in creating that original signal to produce an erection.

More about that signal now. The neurophysiological mechanisms involved in the process of arousal can appear so complicated that it sometimes seems like a miracle that *anyone* ever gets an erection. The simplified version goes like this:

The *autonomic* (in other words, not consciously controlled) functions of the body, such as pulse rate and, yes, erections, are controlled by two parts of the nervous system called sympathetic and parasympathetic. The sympathetic system is responsible for charging the body for "fight or flight" action, such as making the heart beat faster and increasing oxygen intake. The parasympathetic system is then responsible for relaxing the body after the event has passed.

And this is where the paradox lies. Remember how we learned that, for an erection to occur, the smooth muscle in the penis, which is normally contracted, must *relax* in order to let blood in? This means that, while your heart may race and your breath quicken at the prospect of a sexual encounter (all triggered by the sympathetic nervous system), it is actually the *parasympathetic* nervous system that must respond to tell your penis to relax and let the blood in. No wonder we sometimes get our signals crossed! And no wonder that the best sexual experiences usually occur in relaxed, comfortable situations.

The brain and spinal cord work in concert to produce an erection. The brain acts on erotic thoughts, visual stimulus, or mental images (psychogenic erections), while the spinal cord responds to direct touch (reflexogenic erections). This reflex action is assisted by the male hormone testosterone, and by brain messengers called neurotransmitters. In recent years, advances in molecular biology have resulted in signifiant improvements in our understanding of the cellular mediators responsible for the smooth muscle relaxation necessary for erections to take place.

Under normal, nonaroused conditions, a man's sympathetic nervous system sends the neurotransmitter noradrenaline to his penis, which causes the smooth muscle tissue to remain contracted. When a man becomes aroused, the sympathetic nerves are inhibited and the parasympathetic nerves activate, sending the neurotransmitter nitric oxide (NO) to the penis. NO does not act directly, but instead works through a chemical intermediary called cyclic guanosine monophosphate (cGMP). It is cGMP that initiates the muscular and vascular changes that lead to an erection.

And this is where Viagra comes in. There is an enzyme called phosphodiesterase 5 (PDE-5) that is found primarily in the penis. Its job is to break down cGMP. While it does this all the time, during a healthy erection enough cGMP is active, relaxing smooth muscle cells and allowing blood to enter, that the PDE-5 has little effect. Once the nervous system is no longer sending the signal, via nitric oxide, for an erection (after ejaculation, or due to some disruption), PDE-5 breaks down the cGMP, which then can't make the smooth muscle cells relax, and they automatically contract. Viagra works by blocking PDE-5's effect on cGMP. So with nothing inactivating cGMP, it is able to stay in the penis longer (hence longer erections) and at higher levels (hence more fully relaxed smooth muscle and fuller, harder erections). This is why Viagra does not cause erections in the absence of a sexual stimulus: it does not create a sexual signal, but only blocks the mechanism that usually reduces erections.

TYPES OF ERECTILE DYSFUNCTION

As can be seen from the above anatomical sketch, a whole lot must go right for an erection to occur, and the areas where a problem may arise are many. The

CAUSES OF ERECTILE DYSFUNCTION

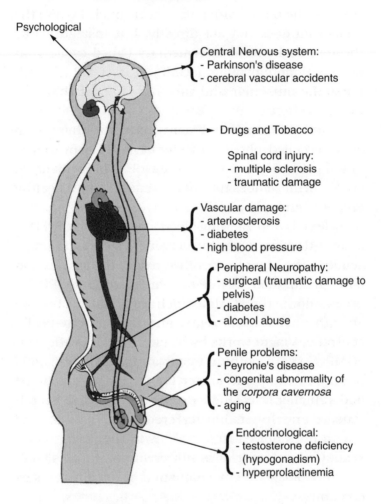

Psychological

Central Nervous system:
- Parkinson's disease
- cerebral vascular accidents

Drugs and Tobacco

Spinal cord injury:
- multiple sclerosis
- traumatic damage

Vascular damage:
- arteriosclerosis
- diabetes
- high blood pressure

Peripheral Neuropathy:
- surgical (traumatic damage to pelvis)
- diabetes
- alcohol abuse

Penile problems:
- Peyronie's disease
- congenital abnormality of the *corpora cavernosa*
- aging

Endocrinological:
- testosterone deficiency (hypogonadism)
- hyperprolactinemia

brain may not produce the right signal (psychological or endocrinological problems), or the signal may not trigger the proper reaction by the penis (neurological problems), or all that may go right but the penis simply won't fill with blood and stay inflated (vascular problems). These problems are in turn caused by a host of conditions, behaviors, injuries, and diseases. Let's examine each.

ENDOCRINAL CAUSES

The endocrine system of glands is responsible for releasing hormones into the body. The primary hormone associated with male sexuality is testosterone. Low testosterone levels in the body have been associated with reduced sex drive, however, testosterone has practically no effect on the physical conditions of erection. Hormonal testosterone treatment for erectile dysfunction is only indicated in patients with low levels of testosterone, and even then it has not proven to be terribly effective in reestablishing erections. In the past, testosterone has been overprescribed for erectile dysfunction not related to hormonal deficiencies.

Another endocrinological problem connected to sexual dysfunction is hyperprolactinemia, the oversecretion of prolactin by the pituitary gland. This is often caused by a pituitary adenoma (a benign tumor). Doctors are often alerted to this condition by signs of gynecomastia (swelling of the breast tissue in men) or the lack of development of the testicles. Hyperprolactinemia is entirely treatable.

While diabetes is a disease of the endocrine system (the body fails to produce sufficient insulin to metabolize food properly), it causes erectile dysfuntion by affecting the vascular and nervous systems. Diabetes causes scarring to build up in the arteries, meaning that they have less space to transport blood and are less elastic, unable to fully dilate during an erection to handle the increased blood flow. Diabetes also damages the nerve endings of the penis. It is the most common cause of erectile dysfunction: 50 percent of all male diabetics will have ED at some stage in their lives. The good news is that diabetes-related ED is usually treatable with substances that improve blood flow to the penis. A simple check for diabetes by testing the blood and urine should be automatic in all ED cases.

Vascular Causes

Blockage of the arteries carrying blood to the penis is the most common cause of physical (as opposed to psychological) erectile dysfunction. It can be caused by diabetes or by all the same factors that increase the risk of heart attack—anything that tends to cause blockages in the blood vessels that lead to the heart will do the same in the blood vessels leading to the penis. Smoking, excessive alcohol consumption, a sedentary lifestyle, and a diet high in cholesterol and saturated fat, or low in "good" high-density lipoprotein (HDL) cholesterol, all contribute to atherosclerosis (hardening of the arteries). In these cases, the resulting erectile dysfunction can be symptomatic of a much more serious problem. A responsible health care practitioner will not simply prescribe Viagra in such cases, which might produce an erection, despite the impeded blood supply, but would do nothing to remedy the possibly life-threatening blockage of the arteries around the heart. A healthy, low-fat diet, regular exercise, quitting smoking, and moderate drinking will usually bring about the return of natural erections, as well as increased life expectancy.

In rare cases, there may be a block in the blood

supply to the penis not connected to atherosclerosis. Generally this is the result of damage to the pelvis. In these instances, revascularization surgery can be performed to bypass the blockage by transferring a blood vessel from beneath the abdominal muscle and connecting it to the penile artery. This procedure is usually reserved for younger men who do not show signs of atherosclerosis. In rare cases where a specific arterial lesion is suspected, arteriography (a radiological procedure in which x-ray-sensitive "dye" is introduced into the arteries) can be considered with a view toward reconstructive surgery.

Hypertension (high blood pressure) is another common vascular cause of erectile dysfunction. Here, it is not buildup of cholesterol in the walls of the arteries that is the problem, but simply constriction of the blood vessels, though the result is the same— less blood is able to move through the system.

One cause of vascular ED that until recently was little known is bicycling. While the cardiovascular benefits of serious cycling are a big health benefit, it seems that the tremendous pressure concentrated on the penile artery by those pointy bicycle seats can cause ED in those men who log serious miles on their bikes each year. This phenomenon has been an unspoken secret in the competitive cycling world and only came to light in the last year or so, despite the fact that some doctors estimate that more than 100,000 American men have been left permanently impotent from cycling. New bicycle seats that spread pressure to other areas of the pelvis are now on the market, and it is my hope that all concerned cyclists will try them out.

If an individual is able to achieve erection normally, but then quickly loses it, we know that the problem is not with the arteries but rather that other half of the circulatory system—the veins. As we all recall from our first biology class, the arteries carry blood from the heart to the body, and the veins return the oxygen-depleted blood to the heart. As we discussed previously, for an erection to occur blood must reach the penis and be trapped there, and this trapping is accomplished by the swelling corpora cavernosa pinching off the veins against the tunica albuginea. In a venous leakage disorder, this pinching off is not completely successful, and blood slips out of the penis and back into the general blood supply, causing the erection to "deflate" just like a leaking tire. Doppler ultra sonography (color flow doppler ultrasound) can help to reveal blood flow through the penis and determine if this is the problem. This form of vascular ED is much rarer than the arterial form.

NEUROLOGICAL CAUSES

The sex act is governed by the whole nervous system. It follows that any cause which might affect the balance of that system can lead to erectile dysfunction. Diabetes can provoke neurological damage leading to erectile dysfunction, as can alcoholism. Multiple sclerosis, Parkinson's disease, polio, cerebral vascular accidents, brain tumors, and traumas of the spinal cord can all prevent the necessary signals from reaching the penis. Neurologic examination should focus on penile sensation, bubble cavernous reflex, anal sphincter tone, and perineal sensation.

Certain operations in the urogenital area, particularly those for prostate or colorectal cancer, may generate erectile dysfunction through damage to peripheral nerves. Of course, the reality of facing cancer is a great emotional strain that can itself induce depression with the symptom of erectile dysfunction. As with so many types of ED, it can be very difficult to try to determine where the physical causes stop and the psychological ones begin.

PEYRONIE'S DISEASE

Peyronie's disease is a naturally occurring condition, the symptoms of which can also result from intracavernous injections. In 1743 François Gigot de la Peyronie, Louis XV's surgeon, was the first to identify this disease of the penis now named after him. As its Latin denomination, *induratio penis plastica*, indicates, the pathology of this disease involves the appearance of scar tissue (plaque) under the tunica albuginea (the tough elastic sheath of the corpus cavernosum). The scars are a few centimeters wide and sensitive. The erection becomes painful and the penis becomes deformed. The plaque itself is benign, or noncancerous. A plaque on the top of the shaft causes the penis to bend upward; a plaque on the underside causes it to bend downward. In some cases, plaque develops on both top and bottom, leading to shortening of the penis. At times, pain, physical changes, and emotional distress associated with Peyronie's disease prohibit sexual intercourse.

There is some evidence that Peyronie's disease, which occurs in 1 percent of men, is an autoimmune disorder and perhaps hereditary, but the majority of cases are probably the result of trauma. The initial accident may be minor, but as the injury heals, scar tissue forms and deformation results. Although the disease occurs mostly in middle-aged men, younger and older men can acquire it. Because the plaque of Peyronie's disease often shrinks or disappears without treatment, medical experts suggest waiting two or more years before attempting to correct it surgically. Some researchers have administered vitamin E orally to men with Peyronie's disease and have reported improvements. Ultrasound therapy on the penis can also speed up the disappearance of the plaque.

Pharmaceutical Causes

Though not easily defined as vascular, endocrinological, or nervous in function, drugs—including alcohol and nicotine—are among the most frequent causes of erectile dysfunction. Alcohol is a classic depressant, which means it has a sedative effect on the nervous system. This is not a problem after one or two drinks—in fact many people find that moderate drinking helps them to relax, forget the day, and get in a romantic mood—but excessive drinking can lead to impairment of both motor functions and the autonomic nervous sytem, making an erection impossible.

And though every Hollywood movie seems to feature characters smoking before and after (and sometimes during!) lovemaking, the truth is that nicotine clogs arteries and constricts blood vessels, restricting function of some things you might want to keep around—like your head, heart, and penis.

The number of prescription and over-the-counter drugs that can be responsible for ED is dizzying, and underlines just how delicate a psychosomatic event erection is. Some of the drugs that commonly cause erectile problems include:

- H_2 antagonist antacids, used to relieve ulcers: cimetidine, ranitidine, and famotidine
- psychotropic drugs, including anxiolytics, sedative-hypnotics, neuroleptics, antiepileptics, antidepressants, mood stabilizers, and appetite suppressants
- high blood pressure medications
- anticholesterol drugs
- diuretics
- cardiac medication
- chemotherapy drugs
- antiandrogens

Drugs used to treat depression are a common cause of erectile dysfunction, and these situations are particularly confusing, because depression alone can cause ED, as well as the other way around. If the patient's erectile dysfunction is the source of the depression, obviously treating the depression with drugs will do no more than at best temporarily lift the depression. The patient may feel better for a week or two, but if he is still not sexually functioning the depression is sure to return. However, it is important to stress that the depression is the far more dangerous condition of the two, as far as the patient's life is concerned, so it is vital that the depression be addressed immediately and not go untreated, even if this means delaying ED treatment.

Conversely, there are depressed patients who are given antidepressants that have a sexual side effect (decreased libido, impaired ejaculation, or difficulty in getting or maintaining an erection). The patient may recover from his depression at first, but then the new sexual problem caused by the medication may trigger fresh anxiety. Worse, if the antidepressant prevents him from feeling appropriately upset by his erectile difficulties and dealing with those feelings, it could result in serious psychological difficulties.

In these delicate situations, the choice of drug is very important. Clinical research has shown that for some patients taking the antidepressant medications known as Selective Serotonin Reuptake Inhibitors (SSRIs), a partial drug holiday of two or three days can help those experiencing sexual dysfunction as a side-effect. Drug holidays, regular periods in which the patient does not take medication, may allow for significant improvement in sexual functioning without a significant return of depressive symptoms. Brief drug holidays may, therefore, provide a practical alternative to additional medication for some patients. There is also some evidence that ginkgo biloba can reverse the sexually inhibiting side-effects of the SSRIs.

Quality of life has become an increasingly important issue in the treatment of depression, and the search for new antidepressant drugs that have less effect on sexuality has gained steam in recent years. Mirtazapine, bupropion, nefazodone, tianeptine, and moclobemide all have little or no impact on sexual function. The physician should, if possible, prescribe one of those medications if it is necessary to treat depression in conjunction with sexual dysfunction.

PSYCHOLOGICAL CAUSES

Causes of psychological impotence are so numerous, varied, and individual that it is impossible to list them all, but most frequently these cases are connected to depression, performance anxiety, marital stress, or mental illness. Depression-related ED can be particularly tricky to treat, because so many of the drugs prescribed to treat depression actually cause erectile dysfunction, and because the onset of erectile dysfunction can certainly cause depression. Determining whether the chicken or the egg came first can be difficult.

Other than mental illness, all the forms of psychological ED are frequently linked to the changes in a man's life that generally occur in his forties or fifties. His body begins to exhibit real signs of aging. He gains weight, loses hair, and wrinkles begin to appear on his face. Suddenly his body, which has always been something he could count on and was even proud of, becomes a source of worry and embarassment. He begins to think of himself in a new way.

Health problems often arise at this time as well, sometimes in conjunction with bad habits that have either been established for some time but previously had little effect (such as a poor diet, or overconsumption of alcohol or tobacco), or become newly established due to aging factors, such as in the case of a man who has been physically active his whole life but slowly finds himself no longer exercising.

Often a man's children are young adults no longer living at home, and they have begun their own sexual lives. In fact, in all likelihood they are now more sexually active than their father. All of this reminds the man of his own youthful sexuality, which, it becomes clearer than ever, is now gone.

A man's working life often changes at this time as well. Younger men with newer skills or technical knowledge may assume more central roles in his company. He may be laid off or moved to a less prestigious position that carries with it fewer responsibilities and a lower salary. He may perhaps find himself having to exchange his house or car for something less expensive, and hence smaller. No matter how well he handles it, this is a terribly threatening challenge to his social status. And, despite decades of "liberation," social status is as important to most men as it always has been. For every primate, as well as most other mammals, social status is a key issue in life. And we are no exception. No wonder then that, confronted by the customary stereotypes of a man's role in society and coming up short, men in this situation often exhibit symptoms of depression, and one of the more common ways for this depression to manifest itself is in erectile dysfunction—in fact, ED is almost twice as prevalent in men suffering from depression as it is in other men.

In contrast to the man, his wife, free of child-care duties for the first time in years, can begin to devote herself to her own professional life. She already has her status as a mother, and now has the opportunity to earn her own money and have professional responsibilities as well. Her partner may find this a difficult situation to adjust to, seeing it as yet another challenge to his status as the breadwinner.

The aging of the sex drive of men and women also appears to be disproportionate. Women often find menopause sexually liberating, whereas for men erectile capabilities generally peak in their twenties or thirties.

Sexual intercourse represents for a man a moment of profound exchange with his partner, and the inability to produce an erection for the purpose may be perceived by him as more than a mere physical failing. He experiences this as a defeat that generates feelings of insecurity, self-doubt, and shame, often linked to feelings of guilt. He no longer feels capable of satisfying his partner. His anguish can be unbearable. This anxiety takes up all his time, and he may begin to "watch" himself during sexual relations in order to attempt mentally to control his erections. This reinforced vigilance normally only aggravates erectile difficulty.

The patient exhibiting erectile dysfunction no longer has a sexuality governed by the search for pleasure. The sexual act becomes a performance undertaken in order to restore his virile identity—a self-test. Thus begins the vicious circle of performance anxiety. The man is anxious about performing and fears a fresh failure measured by the ideal standard he has set up for himself. This anxiety, of course, makes it all the harder for him to perform well, leading to another failure. And this new failure further increases his anxiety, making it even more difficult for him to perform naturally. (The biological explanation for this is that an episode of stress has triggered a predominant number of sympathetic neurotransmitters—the fight or flight response—which inhibit erection, as explained earlier in this chapter.)

Performance anxiety is a problem in itself, but it can also manifest as a decrease in desire. This is not any loss in direct sexual drive, but rather a situation in which the man begins to dread the prospect of arousing his partner for fear of being unable to satisfy her. He then starts avoiding all physical contact and demonstrations of affection. Any intimate situation that carries the risk of leading to sex is avoided. Because of his feelings of guilt and shame, the man doesn't verbally explain to his partner the reasons for this change in his behavior. This absence of communication leads to misunderstandings that further erode the relationship. The woman feels neglected, ignored, and imagines that she is no longer loved, or even that her husband is cheating on her. She can react with anger, jealousy, and may even avoid, in her turn, sexual relations that are frustrating her. All of this only increases the tension between the couple and reinforces performance anxiety by attaching too much symbolism to intercourse and thereby making it a huge psychological barrier. It is in this way that a minor erectile problem of one or two evenings (caused by something as simple as fatigue) can turn into chronic erectile dysfunction.

If the situation reaches this stage, it is obvious that Viagra or any other treatment to simply restore erectile capability will do little to solve the problem. Consulting a sex therapist is the best way to assure that all emotional issues are addressed and that both people involved are ready to reestablish healthy, loving sexual relations. See chapter 10 of this book for an in-depth discussion of how sex therapy works, who it is appropriate for, and what can be gained from it.

Problems relating to loss of erectile capability due to depression or identity problems should not be confused with andropausis, more commonly known as male menopause. To what extent andropausis is a physical change, rather than a psychological one, is a controversial subject in the medical field. Sexual intercourse can certainly take place until a very advanced age. And, as has been discussed, retirement from active work can involve a radical reorganization of a couple's physical relationship. But it is clear that physiological changes *do* affect an aging man's sexuality. Libido and erotic desires are still present but express themselves less intensely. Sexual activity slows down. Spontaneous nocturnal erections are less frequent. An erection takes longer to manifest itself under erotic stimuli and is less reliable for prolonged sexual intercourse. Ejaculation takes longer to achieve, and sexual intercourse often does not lead to ejaculation. The ejaculation is not as powerful as it used to be and the volume of sperm dwindles. Orgasm is less intense. The length of time it takes to achieve an erection after having had one becomes longer.

Most men do not experience any significant modification in their testosterone levels as they grow older. However, if sexual activity becomes rare after sixty, there is a progressive lowering of the testosterone level in the blood. This is definitely a manifestation of andropausis, explained by a weaker vascularization of the testicles. Use it or lose it, guys! Many men over sixty who, for whatever reasons, experience a period of abstinence give up sex for the rest of their lives. In addition, cardiovascular and prostate disorders become common in elderly men and often require treatments that can lead to erectile dysfunction. As far as the physiology of the penis is concerned, some men will age before others with respect to their collagen (the smooth muscle tissue in the penis), a loss of elasticity resulting in an increasingly less rigid erection. This process is irreversible.

Nevertheless, many men who are in good health and happy with their partners continue to have very satisfactory sexual relationships in spite of the aging process. It may be that such men retain a kind of cognitive youth, a state of mind that encourages normal sexuality and dynamism in their everyday life.

To determine if erectile dysfunction is truly psychological, it can be helpful to monitor a man's nocturnal erections. These occur during REM (rapid eye movement) sleep, of which the average man has four or five episodes per night. REM sleep is also called paradoxical sleep because, while one is deeply asleep, the cerebral cortex, the center of higher brain functions, is active in a way that resembles waking consciousness. The eyes dart back and forth rapidly and the breathing grows irregular, but most other muscle activity is inhibited (probably as a safety mechanism). It is in this phase of sleep that dreams occur.

During REM sleep, healthy males experience erections as well as rapid eye movements. Erections begin even before birth, in the mother's uterus. A male fetus already has reflex erections during his phases of REM sleep, and these will continue on a physiological level until death. Each erection occurs about ninety minutes apart.

These erections generally have little to do with erotic dreams. Instead, they are due to activity in the sympathetic and parasympathetic nervous systems located in the spinal cord. In short, erections of this kind are spontaneous and involuntary (reflexogenic) and not psychologically prompted. Doctors have speculated on the role played by nocturnal erections. It seems likely that they help to maintain a healthy penis by periodically flushing the erectile tissue with fresh blood rich in oxygen.

Because nocturnal erections are autonomic, and not triggered by any conscious brain activity, they can be very useful in determining the cause of a man's erectile dysfunction. If a man with ED can still have normal nocturnal erections—if the penis is satisfactorily hard and the erection lasts for several minutes—then there is no question that the penis is functioning correctly as an organ, and we can rule out any physiological cause. It follows that the erectile dysfunction must have a psychological origin—a mental block that is preventing the usual functioning of the penis during sexual intercourse. As a general rule, psychological erectile dysfunction makes its appearance suddenly, out of the blue, while physiological erectile dysfunction creeps up stealthily and by degrees.

PENIS SIZE

And now a word about penis size. I hesitate to even bring up this subject, because rarely has there been such a waste of energy as in the time that men through the ages have spent worrying about the size of their member. As any enlightened lover knows, good sex has everything to do with emotional closeness, setting, and technique, and nothing to do with mass. Still the myth persists—beginning with prepubescent boys and filtering right up to little-boy men—that size matters, and this myth has caused a great deal of psychological turmoil for men. So, in the interest of eliminating ignorance, here are the facts.

Despite the increased availability of sexual information, many people are still woefully ignorant about penis size. Films such as *Boogie Nights*, in which the star Mark Wahlberg was fitted with a huge prosthetic penis, do not help matters. What is normal? Eight inches for an erect penis? Ten?

Actually, the average length of a man's erect penis is between five and six inches, and the average diameter is about an inch and a half at its widest place. The size of the erect penis is relatively unrelated to the size of the flaccid penis. Since only about four inches are needed for satisfactory penetration of the vagina, the number of men who are not adequately equipped for good sex is very small. With the aging process, the penis can lose 0.4 to 0.8 inches in length through gradual fibrosis of the tissues. Elastin and other connective body fibers become progressively replaced by less elastic collagen.

There is absolutely no relationship between penis size and stature, hand size, nose size, or any other body part size. Penis size is purely a matter of genetics and heredity.

Compared to other primates, man has far and away the largest penis and testicles, relative to body size. This is not mere coincidence: as man developed an upright gait, the penis was no longer concealed beneath the body and became an important sexual display, signaling virility to females, much like the red throats on frigate birds or the antlers on deer. With the upright gait came face-to-face intercourse, which allowed for a snug fit of penis in vagina and thus triggered the evolution of the hydraulics that create erections—as well as erectile dysfunction!—in the human male. Most other primates have spiny projections on the glans of their penises that help to anchor the penis in the vagina, while many other mammals, such as dogs, have a penis with an inner bone, known as an os penis, making penetration a simpler affair. In terms of length, man's 5–6 inches beats the gorilla's 3 inches and the orangutang's 1.5 inches hands down, but comes up far short of the bear's 18 inches, the horse's 30, the elephant's 80, and most assuredly the blue whale's 96 inches, or 8 feet.

Interestingly, though the modern Western world believes that large penises are to be desired, this has not always been the case. The ancient Greeks considered the masculine ideal to be a young man with a very small penis and firm, well-muscled buttocks. This explains why so many classical statues of heroes exhibit these characteristics—notably Michelangelo's *David*. A large penis and flabby buttocks were, for the Greeks, signs of lechery; these characteristics were reserved for images of debauchers, barbarians, slaves, and, of course, satyrs.

If a man displays too much anxiety about the size of his penis, recourse to a psychologist or psychiatrist may be necessary. The problem doesn't lie with the size of the penis; what requires treatment is the anxiety that has fixated itself on the theme of size. Often when a man is exhibiting a problem obtaining or maintaining an erection, an anxiety concerning penis size can manifest itself.

PENIS ENLARGEMENT

Oh, the lengths to which men will go! Though it has no effect on sexual performance, this has not stopped men from attempting to enlarge their penises—both in the past and the present day. Let's take a look at some of these ghastly practices, if for no other reason than to underscore just how fixated on penis size some men may be.

The Kama Sutra, the fourth-century Hindu love manual, is perhaps the oldest text to discuss penis enlargement. It offers this agonizing recipe:

> First rub your penis with wasp stings,
>> and massage it with sweet oil.
> When it swells, let it dangle for ten nights
>> through a hole in your bed,
>> going to sleep each night on your stomach.
> After this period use a cool ointment
>> to remove the pain and swelling.
> By this method men of insatiable sexual appetite
>> manage to keep their lingams enlarged
>> throughout their lives.

Before rushing to the nearest wasp's nest, you may want to check out the treatments found in *The Perfumed Garden,* a sixteenth-century Arabic volume that reveals the mysteries of eros:

A man, therefore, with a small member, who
wants to make it grand or fortify it for coitus,
must rub it before copulation with tepid water,
until it gets red and extended by the blood
flowing into it, in consequence of the heat; he
must then anoint it with a mixture of honey and
ginger, rubbing it in sedulously.

Another remedy consists in a compound
made of a moderate quantity of pepper, lavender,
galanga, and musk, reduced to powder, sifted,
and mixed up with honey and preserved ginger.
The member, after having been first washed in
warm water, is then vigorously rubbed with the
mixture; it will then grow large and brawny.

A third remedy is the following: wash the
member in water until it becomes red, and
enters into erection. Then take a piece of soft
leather, upon which is spread hot pitch, and
envelop the member with it. It will not be long
before the member raises its head, trembling
with passion. The leather is to be left on until the
pitch grows cold and the member is again in a
state of repose. This operation, several times
repeated, will have the effect of making the
member strong and thick.

Another way is to bruise leeches with oil,
and rub the member with this ointment; or, if it
is preferred, the leeches may be put into a bottle,
and, thus enclosed, buried in a warm dung-hill
until they are dissolved into a coherent mass
and form a sort of liniment, which is used for
repeatedly anointing the member. The member is
certain greatly to benefit by this.

For another procedure I will here note the
use of an ass's member. Procure one and boil it,
together with onions and a large quantity of
corn. With this dish feed fowls, which you eat
afterward. One can also macerate the ass's verge
in oil, and use the fluid thus obtained for anointing one's member, and drinking of it.

Not to be outdone by the ancients, modern medicine
has invented equally gothic methods of enlarging the
penis.

The Bihari procedure, developed in the 1960s
by an Egyptian doctor, consists of cuting the ligament that secures the base of the penis to the body.
The procedure is dependent on the fact that a man's
penis extends back into his body, beyond what can
be seen externally, and attaches to the pubic bone.
This anchors the erect penis, allowing for control and
support. No actual extra length is created by the Bihari
procedure; instead, 0.5–2 inches of the internal penis is simply made external, creating the impression
of increased length and making it possible to penetrate slightly deeper into the vagina.

The trade-off for this is immense, however. Because the penis is no longer anchored to the body, its
erection no longer stands firm but weaves about, and
during sexual intercourse the man must direct his
penis to its objective with his hand. Sex may not be
resumed following surgery for three to four weeks,
and it takes three to six months to achieve maximum
erection length. Most important, postoperative
stretching and the use of weights are essential to prevent reattachment of the suspensory ligament to the

penis.It seems very unlikely that satisfactory sex can be achieved by undergoing this method, which costs about $3,000 to $4,500.

Fat injection (or lipotransfer method) is the process of removing fat from the back of the thighs and injecting it into the body of the penis, thereby thickening it. Because the body rejects a significant portion of the injection, this procedure may need to be repeated several times and each operation carries with it a risk of infection. Because the penile shaft is narrower than the maximum diameter of the head, the doctor usually fills out the shaft only slightly beyond the head's maximum diameter to maintain proper proportions. In this operation circumference can be increased by 50 percent or more. Sexual activity can usually be resumed within two weeks, but the long-term risks of fat injection remain uncertain. The procedure costs $4,500 to $7,000.

Dermal grafting is an alternative procedure to increase penile girth. The results appear to be more permanent and the penis can be made much thicker than with the lipotransfer method. In this procedure, two strips of fat are taken from the back of the thighs and are implanted on either side of the penis. The surgeon cuts down to the layer of tissue known as Buck's fascia. The outer layers of the penile skin are then separated from Buck's fascia, and the fat strips are grafted onto it. The skin incisions are then sewed back together.

More recently, in June 1999 doctors in Shaghai successfully reconstructed the penises of two men who had lost theirs, one to amputation due to a tumor and one to an accident. The doctors used skin and muscle from the patients' thighs, stomach, and forearms, and claim that nerve sensation is restored as well. Both men were able to father children after recovery.

Obviously, penile lengthening operations in normal patients remain a major question, and the above procedures are quite controversial. Surgeons who perform them feel that they should only be prescribed for those few men who really do have penises small enough to be considered sexually handicapped—usually less than three inches when erect. Psychiatric consultation is necessary for an evaluation of the patient's motivations and expectations.

3 BEFORE VIAGRA

OTHER ALLOPATHIC
TREATMENTS FOR ED

Before Viagra came along you rarely heard the word "impotence" being mentioned in public, much less "erectile dysfunction," but that doesn't mean that the problem wasn't out there. Erectile dysfunction has tormented men throughout history. The nineteen-thousand-year-old cave paintings at Lascaux in France depict rituals for averting and treating an erectile disorder, and the ancient Egyptian myth of Osiris—in which the god was dismembered into fourteen pieces and, when reassembled, was missing his penis, and could not come back to life until a new penis was found and "animated" by the mouth of his wife, Isis—is a clear allegory of erectile dysfunction and fertility. In the Middle Ages ED was commonly held to be the work of the devil and his human servants, who would cast spells on the bridegroom during the wedding ceremony, and a standard part of the service was the priest's threat of excommunication of any who tried.

In the twentieth century ED is more widespread than ever, and doctors have spent a great deal of effort searching for a cure. Though the purpose of this book is to examine the pros and cons of Viagra and to present a range of healthier, more holistic ways of overcoming ED, we should still take a brief look at the other allopathic methods for treating ED. There are two reasons for doing this: one, to give you an idea of how horrific the state of ED treatments was before Viagra, which will help you to understand why Viagra was hailed as revolutionary, but will also make it that much more perplexing why readily available and far more appealing holistic remedies were not more sought out. The second reason for surveying these techniques is because there are still a minority of men who don't respond to psychotherapeutic treatments, alternative remedies, or Viagra, and who find that these older medical treatments are the only options open to them.

Twenty years ago sexual problems were not generally taught to doctors at medical school. The treatment of erectile dysfunction has traditionally been considered the domain of urologists, psychiatrists, and psychologists. General practitioners routinely sent patients with sexual difficulties to psychiatrists. Prior to 1983, clinicians had limited therapeutic options available for alleviating erectile dysfunction. Vacuum constriction devices, penile prosthetic implants, and hormone replacement therapy were the chief alternatives for physical conditions, while psychotherapy was the treatment of choice for psychogenic dysfunctions.

In 1969, in *Everything You Always Wanted to Know about Sex but Were Afraid to Ask*, David R.

Reuben, M.D., stated, "There is convincing evidence that the source of male potency is in the brain." This illustrates the "all-in-the head" theories of the past. Until fairly recently it was believed that the majority of cases of erectile dysfunction had psychological roots. Now, with the identification of neurotransmitters in the penis, and the Viagra gold rush on, it is believed that 80 percent of ED cases have physiological roots. The truth probably lies somewhere in the middle. This is a classic case of official "beliefs" being customized to point to the dominant modality: When physiological treatments rarely worked, it was believed that most ED cases were psychological in origin, but now that doctors are having success with vacuum constriction devices, penile injection therapy, and Viagra, it is to their advantage to believe that most cases are physical in origin.

Before we examine each device in turn, I should let you in on a little secret that the doctors and manufacturers won't tell you. When you hear the statistics for men achieving erections with these methods, they sound pretty successful. But what is left out is the fact that these restored erections often did not lead to restored intercourse, either because the couples could not get past the awkwardness and clunkiness of the devices, which ruined the spontaneity of sex, or because the underlying emotional issues that had caused the ED in the first place were still unresolved.

THE EVALUATION

Before choosing a course of action for ED treatment, the physician will conduct a full physical examination of the patient, along with a thorough medical and sexual history. This is very important, even for men who plan to treat their ED themselves through herbs, supplements, or lifestyle changes, because it can uncover life-threatening health conditions.

While it can be difficult to answer some very frank questions, the sexual history is the single most useful part of the evaluation. The patient should not interpret these questions as intrusive, and must be equally frank with his responses if he expects to obtain help. Questions may well include some or most of the following:

- Do you currently have erections?
- Are your erections straight or curved?
- Do you have erections at night?
- When was the last time you had a full, rigid erection?
- Do you ever awaken with erections in the morning?
- When was the last time you had sexual intercourse? Did you penetrate? Did you ejaculate? Did your partner climax?
- Do you achieve an erection but lose it before or soon after beginning intercourse?
- Does the quality or duration of your erection vary at times or with different sexual partners?
- Do you have any concern regarding the size of your penis?
- Are you able to achieve a climax or an orgasm? If so, how is this achieved? Vaginal? Manual? Oral? Anal?

- Does semen come out the end of your penis when you have an orgasm?
- Can you masturbate to climax? If so, does your penis get hard at this time?
- Do you now have or have you ever had premature ejaculations?
- Does reaching a climax seem to take a long time?
- Is your orgasm ever painful?
- Is sensation in your penis normal?
- Do you think that your level of interest in sexual relations is less than most men of your age?
- What is your partner's level of interest in sex?
- Do you believe that your partner contributes to your sexual problem?
- How would you describe the quality of your sexual relationship?
- Is your partner interested in having your sexual problem treated?

The medical history will address medications currently being taken by the patient, along with use of tobacco, alcohol, and recreational drugs. Level of fitness, history of illness, and any other physical problems should be discussed. A psychological profile will explore stress levels related to depression, stressful job situations, impending divorce or separation, and any other life factors.

The physical examination will include examination of the genitalia for elasticity and for the detection of plaquelike formations that would indicate Peyronie's disease. The size and location of the testicles will be noted, along with the presence or absence of masses and hernias. A digital rectal examination of the prostate will be done to assess anal sphincter tone. The physician will also look for abnormal secondary sex characteristics, such as body and facial hair, which could point to hormonal problems.

If the physician suspects that more serious problems may be at the root of the ED, he may do additional laboratory tests. Tests for systemic diseases include blood counts, urinalysis, lipid profile, glucose tolerance tests, and measurements of creatinine and liver enzymes. Measurements of testosterone and prolactin in the blood can yield information about problems with the endocrine system.

If, after gathering as much information as possible, the physician is convinced that the cause of the ED is physical (and if he is not open to alternative therapies), he will probably choose to put the patient on Viagra, but if the patient is one of the 30 to 50 percent who don't find Viagra satisfactory, the physician will likely recommend one of the following treatment methods.

VACUUM CONSTRICTION DEVICES

With a vacuum constriction device (VCD), a plastic cylinder, which is attached by a tube to a hand pump, is placed over the penis. The hand pump is used to create a vacuum inside the cylinder and, within five to seven minutes, the negative pressure "draws" blood into the penis and fills it, causing an erection that is maintained by placing a tight elastic band or ring around the base of the penis. Sexual intercourse is then possible.

The only side effects of VCDs are local and relate to the band used to maintain the erection. Because it is of necessity tight, the band causes the penis to become congested and cool, and, after about half an hour, painful. So, the band should not be kept in place for longer than thirty minutes. There can be pain at the ring, or the penis can feel frozen. Bruising has been reported, but this can be avoided as long as the negative pressure does not exceed 200 mm of mercury. The pump should have a safety valve to guard against exerting excess pressure.

The rigidity of the erection is average, and 80 percent of patients report satisfaction with this solution to their erectile dysfunction. Ejaculation can be postponed or retarded, and when it does occur it is delivered not out the urethra but into the bladder. This is harmless—and actually the goal of certain Tantric yoga practices!

VCDs are still useful in the case of patients who have had major prostate surgery, the majority of whom do not respond to either Viagra or alternative therapies. Of course, the huge drawback of VCDs is that nothing spoils the mood faster than stopping foreplay, whipping out the vacuum cylinder and pump, and engaging in a five-minute procedure.

VCDs can only be purchased with a medical prescription and are usually at least partially covered by insurance companies. Their cost ranges from $200 to $500. There have been reports of injury from devices bought through catalogs. These devices may lack pressure-release valve or other safety elements, so let your doctor recommend brands before you purchase one.

PENILE PROSTHESES

Implanting prostheses in the penis is an idea that takes its cue from nature: most other vertebrates, including primates and dogs, have a bone in their penises so that they are rigid all the time, and when not "in use" are hidden in a shaft.

The French surgeon Ambroise Paré was the inventor of the first penile implant. During the Second World War surgeons attempted to implant rib cartilage into the penises of men who had lost their testicles in battle. Eventually several disadvantages to using cartilage became apparent, and it was entirely replaced by silicone in the seventies.

The procedure consists of placing silicone rods into the two corpora cavernosa. This is an irreversible procedure: erectile tissue is permanently damaged when these devices are implanted. In 1974 another French surgeon perfected this method by inventing a support with an adjustable rod that made vaginal penetration possible. Though the penis would always be the same size and hardness, it could be bent down during daily life to be somewhat less obtrusive, then bent upward and straightened out for sexual intercourse.

The advantage of semirigid implants is that they are simple to use—no moving parts. Once the initial chance of infection has passed, men with these implants experience few problems. The great disadvantage is that the man equipped with a semirigid implant has a permanent erection, though without the same consistency as an ordinary erect penis.

In 1973 Dr. Brantley Scott of Baylor University invented an inflatable implant consisting of paired cylinders that are surgically inserted inside the corpora cavernosa. These can be expanded to create an erection by filling them with fluid through tubes connecting the cylinders to a reservoir implanted in the lower pelvis. Using his hand, the patient inflates and deflates his penis by means of a pump implanted in his scrotum.

Clearly this is a very complicated device. The big benefit, compared to the semirigid implant, is that when deflated it leaves the penis with a fairly natural flaccid appearance. The drawbacks, besides cost, include the higher chance of mechanical failure.

Penile implants of both kinds should only be a last resort, useful for patients with problems that cannot be cured in any other way, such as irreversible lesions of the corpora cavernosa or Peyronie's disease (serious curvature of the penis). They can only be prescribed by a specialist. There is an adaptation period of a few weeks, especially for the semipermanent implants. Afterward, the implant can be kept for many years without needing to be changed. The surgery to install it lasts one to two hours, depending on the type of implant. Mechanical problems have diminished in recent years because of technological advances.

The cost for a penile implant can be anywhere from $5,000 to $20,000, and insurance coverage is spotty.

VASOACTIVE DRUGS

The first paper on medication-induced erections ap-
peared in 1978. Doctors studying the autonomic nervous system's role in cat bladder function noted that
erections resulted from the infusion of phentolamine,
phenoxybenzamine, terbutaline, and salbutamol. The
next development occurred five years later, when Dr.
Giles Brindley described "cavernosal alpha blockade."
He induced erection by injecting 5 mg of phenoxybenzamine hydrochloride, an alpha blocker, into the
corpora cavernosa. Famously, Dr. Brindley once demonstrated his successful technique at a medical con-
ference by dropping his trousers in front of his as-
tonished colleagues to reveal his erect penis, which
he had injected with phenoxybenzamine. Unfortunately, this drug was painful to inject, slow to produce erection, and resulted in penile enlargement for
up to three days.

In 1980, while performing vascular surgery to
clear clogged arteries, Dr. Ronald Virag* discovered
the effect of papaverine on the penis. After performing a deviation of the epigastric artery, the surgeon,
as usual, injected a small dose of papaverine to dilate
the artery. The immediate result was a prolonged erection in the patient.

Dr. Virag concluded that intracavernous injections of papaverine could induce erections by some-

*Readers will undoubtedly notice the similarity between the names Viagra
and Virag. Because of this situation, Dr. Virag has brought a legal suit against
Pfizer laboratories in order to change the product name in France. He doesn't
want to be associated with Viagra, especially after the bad press the medication has received.

how chemically recreating the effect of the neurotransmitters responsible for erection, without any input from the brain. Subsequently the experiment was repeated with volunteers. The results were announced at a congress in 1982 and published in the *Lancet,* and in 1986 Dr. Virag was awarded a prize by the American Society of Urology.

Since this time major advances have occurred in the understanding of neurotransmitters for intracavernous smooth muscle relaxation and contraction, as well as the function of vascular endothelium cells and their gap junctions, and many drugs causing the same phenomenon have been discovered.

Patients must go through several preliminary sessions with a doctor to test reactions and determine the correct levels of vasoactive medication for each particular case. During an office visit, the physician injects the medication into the patient's penis. The comfort, degree of erection obtained, and time it takes to lose the erection are carefully observed by the doctor. After this test, the exact dosage of the drug is determined.

The doctor will then instruct the patient on the technique of self-injections. A latex cast can be used to practice on. The typical injection of 1 cc of the product with a tiny insulin needle is practically painless; some men describe it as merely a mild pinching sensation. The patient bends his penis to the side, pinches it between thumb and forefinger, then injects the medication into the corpora cavernosa. The substance spreads rapidly inside the penis and, with the help of visual stimulation or light masturbation, an erection takes place roughly fifteen minutes later.

Patients can also use an automatic injector, which hides the complete syringe mechanism in a pen-shaped device so that no needle is visible. When placed against the penis, it automatically triggers the injection. This can be very useful for people who are squeamish about needles, because you never have to actively push the needle in. Many diabetes patients who must inject insulin will be familiar with this device. The Medi-Ject corporation is also currently studying a needle-free injection system, which delivers the drug through the skin of the penis without puncturing it.

Penile injections have to be made into one of the cavernous parts on the upper quarter of the penis. Neither the median line running up the penis nor the lower part can be injected. The superficial veins, easily detectable under the skin of the penis, and the glans must also be avoided.

The intracavernous injection of a vasoactive substance induces an immediate relaxation of the smooth muscle, resulting in increased blood flow and an erection. The erection can last between thirty and ninety minutes. It does not always disappear immediately after ejaculation.

Penile injections have proved effective for treating a variety of forms of physical erectile dysfunction, including cases stemming from spinal cord injury, multiple sclerosis, diabetes, cystectomy, and pelvic trauma. Several other drugs besides papaverine are now used. They fall into two categories: inducers of erection, which trigger completely hard erections, and erection facilitators, or "starters," which induce tumescence—the penis becomes swollen but not hard enough to achieve penetration, and sexual stimulation and the body's natural response are required for the development of a full erection. These latter substances are used in cases of mild erectile dysfunction, because they allow for the libido and, most important, the man's partner, to play a more natural role in the sexual act.

One drawback to penile injection therapy is that the injection is a fairly exacting process. The skin has to be cleaned with disinfectant beforehand. The penis must be bent over sideways. The injection has to be firm and the needle must be entirely inserted in the selected site. The substance is injected slowly; if it does not go in easily, a new site must be chosen. Once the whole amount has been injected, the needle must be rapidly withdrawn. The injection site must then be compressed and rubbed with an antiseptic compress. Obviously this process precludes spontaneous sex.

Fear of the injection may at first induce a natural reflex causing the penis to contract, which makes the procedure more difficult. This can be helped by taking a hot bath or shower beforehand.

Normally, the erection takes place within fifteen minutes of the injection and lasts between fifteen minutes and one hour. The best time to administer the injection, therefore, is before foreplay, to preserve the natural rhythm of intercourse as much as possible.

To avoid potential side effects, there should be no more than one injection per day and two injections per week, with an interval of at least twenty-four hours between each two injections to avoid a cumulative effect. Complications, though rare, can include prolonged erections lasting hours, small fibrous nodules appearing on the site of the injection, hematomas and bruises on the injection site, painful erection (this occurs in 18 percent of cases), and bleeding from the injection site.

When an erection lasts more than a few hours, without sexual stimulation, this is known as priapism, and it is the most serious complication of intracavernous injections. It is relatively frequent (2 to 19 percent of cases) when papaverine is used on its own, and is most frequent with younger subjects partly retaining their erectile function, with neurological patients, and when the problem is not vascular in origin. The condition can vanish spontaneously, but it requires medical attention. The doctor can give an injection of phenylephrine, which acts as an antidote. If that fails, the doctor will inject an alpha stimulant product (adrenaline, clonidin, or cortisone). If the erection still doesn't subside, the cavernous bodies need to be punctured through the glans. This is a medical emergency, and the procedure is performed in order to avoid a thrombosis of the cavernous parts due to blood coagulation. If this occurs, surgical intervention is needed for a draining puncture of the cavernous parts under general anesthetic. The possible result of a delayed treatment of priapism is irreversible erectile dysfunction caused by damage to the cavernous bodies, which would require correction by the surgical implantation of a penile prosthesis.

Papaverine is the substance most often blamed for this type of complication. Significant progress has been achieved with the use of others drugs, such as prostaglandins or moxisylyte, which only very rarely induce priapism.

There is no loss of effectiveness of penile injections with long-term use, however, a man who has been cured of a temporary episode of erectile dysfunction by penile injections may find himself with a psychological dependence on the procedure—he lacks confidence in getting an erection on his own. In this case, he should try to have sex without the drug half of the time. This will allow him to slowly regain his confidence, while not completely curtailing his sexual activities in the meantime, which can cause the psychological problem to worsen.

In cases of predominantly psychological ED, it is perfectly possible to reach a stage at which injections cease to be necessary. Most young patients can have a normal erection again within a year of starting the treatment.

As with Viagra, injections shouldn't change the sex habits a couple had established before the onset of erectile dysfunction. One should always beware of confusing erotic satisfaction and sexual performance—especially with penile injections, where the erection can go on far beyond ejaculation, and beyond what one or both partners desire or find comfortable.

The maximum frequency of injections is twice a week, with an interval of at least twenty-four hours in between. Injections generally cost $5 to $40 per injection.

URETHRAL SUPPOSITORIES

In 1997 doctors began using a new way of delivering vasoactive drugs to the penis, based on the discovery that there is an exchange of blood between the corpus spongiosum and the corpora cavernosa. This means that it is possible to affect the smooth muscle of the corpora cavernosa by introducing a drug via the urethra into the corpus spongiosum.

The Medicated Urethral System for Erection (MUSE) is a transurethral drug delivery system consisting of a prefilled plastic applicator containing a urethral medicated pellet (or suppository) of alprostadil. Early studies found that MUSE was well tolerated and was safe for long-term use, but did not measure its effectiveness. Adverse effects included 29 percent reporting penile pain, 5 percent suffering minor urethral bleeding, and 2 percent having some dizziness.

A study at the Medical College of Georgia found some positive results by combining MUSE with an adjustable penile constriction band to promote blood flow. In this study 77 percent of the men reported successful intercourse, and 69 percent were satisfied with their performance. In their own homes, more than 80 percent of respondents who used MUSE with constriction bands rated sexual intercourse as satisfactory. Some other studies, however, have found that a low percentage of patients found MUSE satisfactory.

MUSE works by delivering the drug alprostadil, in a semisolid urethral pellet, into the urethra. Transurethral absorption is rapid (80 percent of a dose within ten minutes). Local absorption relaxes smooth muscle, resulting in rapid arterial inflow and penile rigidity. The erectile process begins five to ten minutes after application.

The MUSE system consists of a small, disposable plastic applicator, which is simply and comfortably inserted into the end of the penis. Once in place, by gently pushing the button on top of the applicator, a pellet about the size of a grain of rice is delivered directly to the urethra.

MUSE should never be used in cases where there is known hypersensitivity to alprostadil; where there is sickle-cell anemia, thrombocythemia, polycythemia, or multiple myeloma; or where there is abnormal penile anatomy such as urethral stricture, balanitis (infection of the glans), severe hypospadias and curvature, or acute urethritis. In addition, alprostadil has been shown to be embryotoxic, so the use of a condom is necessary during intercourse.

MUSE should not be used more than twice within any twenty-four-hour period. It must be kept in a refrigerator and allowed to warm to room temperature about thirty minutes prior to use.

The side effects of MUSE include mild pain in the penis (reported at least once by one third of patients), vaginal burning or itching in the patients' partners (6 percent), and dizziness (3 percent of patients). Priapism is the most serious side effect reported, but it is extremely rare (about one in five hundred patients).

MUSE is not cheap. One dose costs upward of $20.

4 FUTURE DRUGS

THE NEWEST PILLS

Viagra is only the first wave in the exploding field of oral ED treatments. In response to Viagra's vigorous sales, and perhaps also in the wake of the scare about Viagra's side effects, many companies and research facilities are testing and marketing dietary supplements or pharmaceutical products that also promise to enhance sexual experiences for men. It seems likely that within a few years Viagra may be completely eclipsed by drugs and herbal formulations that offer more reliable results with less risk.

APOMORPHINE

This relative of morphine is taken sublingually (placed under the tongue) and is believed to act through dopamine receptors in the brain. In a study of 236 men with ED and hypertension, dosages of 6 mg of apomorphine produced erections sufficient for inter-course in 63 percent of the patients, versus 33 per-cent for a placebo. The most common side effect was nausea, reported by 14 percent of the patients. Apo-morphine may be a promising treatment for men with ED who cannot take Viagra because of hypertension.

ARGINMAX

ArginMax, in existence since March 1998, has two studies to back its claim to improve men's ability to achieve an erection. Made by the Daily Wellness Com-pany of Mountain View, California, the supplement, which you can buy on the Internet and at 3,000 stores predominantly on the U. S. West Coast, costs approxi-mately $40 to $50 a month to use. This price makes it less expensive than Viagra for those that engage in sex more than once a week—and also means you don't have to carry a pill in your wallet at all times. ArginMax combines the amino acid L-Arginine (see discussion in this chapter), ginseng, and ginkgo plus antioxi-dants, vitamin B complex, and minerals such as zinc and selenium, all of which promote sexual fitness. It is a nonprescription supplement with no reported side effects. Men take six pills a day, in two doses.

As noted, two studies have been completed, and others are in the works. An initial research study de-signed by Dr. Andy Das, an Albany Medical Center urologist, showed that 89 percent of men aged forty to seventy-seven with mild to moderate erectile dysfunc-tion improved their sex lives after taking ArginMax for four weeks. Seventy-five percent reported improved sat-isfaction with their overall sex life. Only a small group of twenty-five men were studied; twenty-one actually completed the study.

The second study, of fifty men with no history of sexual problems, also consisted of a daily dose of ArginMax for four weeks. Ages of these subjects ranged from twenty-three to fifty-four. Eighty percent of these men experienced an improvement in the ability to sustain an erection during intercourse, and the same percentage reported an improvement in their overall enjoyment of sex. These are impressive results, and because of its all-natural ingredients and lack of side effects, ArginMax is a very promising treatment for ED, though more studies are necessary to confirm its effectiveness. A new clinical trial underway targets 150 men with ED who have found Viagra unsatisfactory.

DHEA

The hormone DHEA (dehydroepiandrosterone) may also provide an alternative treatment for erectile dysfunction. At the University of Vienna, Dr. Werner J. Reiter and his colleagues performed a trial including forty patients with erectile dysfunction. They randomly assigned either an inactive placebo or 50 mg of DHEA daily over a period of six months. The patients had normal levels of testosterone and other hormones. Those who took DHEA experienced significant improvement in maintaining an erection after sixteen weeks. No adverse effects were reported. Treatment with DHEA looks promising, but future studies are needed to reveal the working mechanisms of the hormone.

GENE THERAPY

Research is underway involving the introduction of genes responsible for erectile function into the smooth penile muscle tissue of animals. In the future it may be possible to introduce these genes into the penises of men suffering from ED, possibly reversing the natural loss of elasticity in the smooth muscle tissue due to aging. It will be many years, however, before this research reaches fruition.

IC351

A joint venture between Eli Lilly and ICOS corporation, IC351 is an oral PDE-5 inhibitor, like Viagra. In the one significant study completed, an amazing 86 percent of patients reported improved erections. On a scale of 1 to 5, the patients rated their IC351 erections as a 4, on average, compared to a rating of 2 for the placebo. No serious adverse effects were reported.

INDIAN DRUGS

Several Indian pharmaceutical companies are producing formulations containing sildenafil, the active agent in Viagra. One company in particular, Cipla, which has sales depots in Bombay and New Delhi, has applied to the Drugs Controller of India for local marketing approval of the drug, which may be on the Indian market in 2000. The company may also be seeking export to other countries. Some media reports indicate that Cipla is already dispatching its first batch of sildenafil to a South American destination, but the company has not commented about marketing approval in the United States. At the present time these drugs are not approved by the FDA.

L-ARGININE

This is an amino acid that lowers cholesterol and can effectively treat impotency in some men. L-arginine is broken down to nitrous oxide, which relaxes blood vessels in the penis and permits greater blood flow to the penis. Natural sources of this amino acid include fish,beans, and peanuts. The recommended dose is 4 to 8 grams at bedtime.

MELANOTAN-II

An extremely promising alternative ED treatment may be Melanotan-II, a synthetic form of a melanocyte-stimulating hormone tested at the University of Arizona. This drug was being developed as a method for turning people's skin pigment dark and thus preventing the damaging effects of ultraviolet radiation from the sun. It had worked successfully on frogs, and when volunteers were injected with the drug, they also turned darker. But one volunteer reported the onset of a spontaneous erection, leading the researchers to test the drug on ten men with ED. Nine of the subjects sustained an erection after receiving Melanotan-II—including one man who had found Viagra to be ineffective—and the erections lasted more than two hours on average.

According to Hunter Wessells, M.D., the lead researcher in the study, Melanotan-II treats psychological and other forms of ED by stimulating the pathways in the brain and nervous system that trigger erection, rather than by increasing blood flow to the penis. Thus it may prove effective in treating physical and psychological ED, and, unlike Viagra, stimulates libido as well. It also seems to have none of the dangerous side effects of Viagra—a need to stretch was the only one reported—since it does not act directly on the cardiovascular system. These results are very preliminary, and years of testing are still required to ascertain the safety and efficacy of Melanotan-II. Though the studies involved an injection of the drug, future clinical trials will focus on a nasal-spray, eyedrop, or pill form.

NuMAN

NuMAN is the name of an herbal product introduced to the U.S. market in May 1998, but its formula has been used for more than fifty years in China. Peipei Wu Wishnow, Ph.D., founder of Interceuticals of Marblehead, Massachusetts, initiated the sale of NuMAN in this country. A research scientist, Wu Wishnow was born in China where she learned to prepare traditional remedies.

NuMAN consists of eighteen pure, natural Chinese herbs. These nonprescription capsules are based on traditional Chinese medicine (TCM) theories. The practice of this type of medicine began about 5,000 years ago in the Sheng Nung period in China. The TCM approach considers the body a whole entity, with each part inseparable from another. The pills are manufactured in China under Good Manufacturing Practice conditions and sold in the United States in health food stores, pharmacies, or by mail order.

In NuMAN, two active herbs are Wu Wei Zi, a dried fruit, and Yin Yang Huo, a dried plant. The first has a protective effect on the liver and may improve mental functions and antagonize the central convulsive effects of caffeine. It also has a direct stimulating effect on the respiratory center and has a potent sperm-stimulating effect. The second herb, Yin Yang Huo, works primarily on the cardiovascular system. It lowers blood pressure and is reputed to have a sexually stimulating effect on males. It can stimulate development of the prostate, testes, and anus rector muscle. Both herbs are considered relatively nontoxic. Some patients may experience some gastrointestinal disturbances, such as nausea and vomiting, or occasional dryness of the mouth. NuMAN is recommended primarily for men older than forty.

Forty-five New England men recently took part in a marketing survey after taking three twenty-day cycles of the capsules; each cycle was followed by three days without the pills. Forty-five percent of the participants were between forty-one and fifty years of age; five percent were older than seventy-one. Seven parameters were measured: erection length; overall sex life satisfaction; partial or full erections when stimulated; ejaculations occurring at appropriate time; firmness of erections for intercourse; level of sex drive; and felt sex drive.

The results of this survey were thoroughly positive. Seventy percent of the participants stated that the supplement improved either their sexual or urinary functions. Sixty percent said NuMAN improved their sexual functions, and 25 percent, only their urinary functions. Fifty-eight percent said their erections lasted as long as they wished, and 54 percent expressed an overall satisfaction with their sex life. Ninety percent expressed the intention to keep taking the product. No one reported any ill side effects.

A recent survey in China of the product showed that among five thousand men who took the capsules, 95 percent experienced varying degrees of improvement in sexual performance; 75 percent reported high satisfaction. In a small survey group of fifty-six, 85 percent reported improvement in urination patterns. No unpleasant side effects have ever been noted in China after fifty years of the product's use. Ongoing human and animal studies are being performed, although no additional results are yet available. The U.S. study is important because a product that works for Chinese men does not necessarily work for American or European men due to variations in lifestyle, diet, and weight.

The recommended dosage is one 0.9 g capsule taken twice a day, before breakfast and following dinner, for twenty days, followed by a three-day break. Results are cumulative and usually require more than one cycle. For best results, men should repeat three consecutive cycles. After this, one cycle per month should be followed by a ten-day break.

TESTOSTERONE

This naturally occurring hormone is responsible for sex drive in men *and* women, as well as the production of male secondary sex characteristics such as a deep voice and facial hair. There is good evidence that men with abnormally low libidos can increase their sex drive by taking testosterone. More controversial is the claim that men with normal libidos can increase their sex drive by taking the hormone. In any case, testosterone has no effect on erections, only on libido, so it is not applicable for men with true ED. It is available as an injection, a transdermal patch, or a pill, but the pill form is associated with serious liver disease and the injection is associated with other health concerns. The patch is the best delivery system.

Testosterone treatments for men have been used for years. What is new, however, is a 1999 study of fifty-seven women who had lost their sex drive after undergoing hysterectomies, which found that more than half reported an increase in libido while using the testosterone skin patches. Even more encouraging was the fact that the women suffered no additional hot flashes, acne, or hair growth, and no changes in estrogen levels. This is very promising, but more studies will have to be done before we can verify these results.

TOPIGLAN

This gel, being studied at Boston University, contains alprostadil, the same drug commonly used in penile injection therapy and in MUSE urethral suppositories, combined with a patented hydrocarbon that allows the alprostadil to be absorbed through the glans (head) of the penis and to pass into the corpora cavernosa. A study of 114 men with ED who applied Topiglan or a placebo gel to their penises and then watched pornographic films found that within forty-five minutes 69 percent of the men who used Topiglan had erections, versus 20 percent of the placebo group. The only side effect noted so far is a warm sensation on the penis.

TRAZODONE

Trazodone, an antidepressant drug sold under the trade name Desyrel, has been discussed as a treatment for erectile dysfunction for years. Many male patients taking trazodone were found to experience priapism, which led researchers to speculate on its possibilities for treating erectile dysfunction. But, as discussed in chapter 3, priapism can be quite painful and dangerous, and any treatment that involves a large risk of this condition should be avoided if possible. Trazodone is sometimes used in combination with yohimbe. Large-scale, well-controlled studies have not been undertaken and are not expected to be. Another side effect of trazodone is cardiac arrhythmia.

UPRIMA

This apomorphine-based pill, a joint venture between a U.S. corporation and a Japanese drugmaker, is in a race with Vasomax to become the first large-scale pharmaceutical competitor to Viagra. Preliminary test results showed Uprima to relieve ED 61 percent of the time, much higher than Vasomax's 40 percent and on a par with Viagra's results.

VASOMAX

Like Viagra, Vasomax works to improve blood flow to the penis. However, this oral phentolamine doesn't interact with nitrates and may provide the best pharmaceutical alternative for men with heart concerns. This prescription drug is produced by Texas-based Zonagen, which also makes Vasofem, a treatment for female sexual dysfunction. In a recent preliminary study, Vasomax worked for 25 to 40 percent of the male participants.

Vasomax passed its first two U.S. studies in 1998. The first was a placebo-controlled, double-blind study that gave randomized doses of 40 to 80 mg of the oral drug or of a placebo. The second was a placebo-controlled, crossover-designed trial of 40 mg oral phentolamine versus a placebo. Those who participated and began the study with mild ED showed mild to moderate dysfunction at the conclusion of the trial. At doses of 40 and 80 mg, respectively, 51 percent of the men achieved penetration on seventy-five percent of attempts, compared with only 38 percent who received a placebo. At 40 mg, fewer than 3 percent experienced specific adverse reactions other than 8 percent who experienced rhinitis. At 80 mg, fewer than 7 percent experienced any adverse effect other than 18 percent who had rhinitis. Other side effects that have been noted are flushing and mild headaches. Vasomax takes effect in 15 to 30 minutes.

Vasomax has been approved and in use in Mexico since 1998 and is in the midst of the FDA approval process, but in spring 1999 Zonagen announced that it would postpone the review process to allow itself more time to show that the drug works. Summer 2000 is the earliest possible date at which the drug will be available.

VIAGRA

What is Viagra doing in the list of *new* treatments for ED? Well, this isn't so much a new drug as a new method of delivery. Instead of using the pill form of Viagra, researchers at Pfizer and the University of Kentucky are working on a nasal-spray delivery system for Viagra. The advantage of the nasal spray is that it would take effect in five to fifteen minutes, instead of over one hour, as is the case for the oral form of Viagra.

Still another new chapter in the Viagra story will be its use by women. Pfizer is currently performing clinical trials to test Viagra's effectiveness in overcoming women's sexual dysfunctions, and even now doctors are allowed to prescribe Viagra to women and thousands of women are using it. From the research that has been conducted so far, it seems that the male and female sexual systems are not so different as once thought. A woman's clitoris and vagina need to become engorged with blood for a satisfactory sexual experience just as a man's penis does, and Viagra seems to be equally effective for women. Considering that the number of women suffering from sexual problems is even higher than the number of men, in a few years Viagra may be considered primarily a drug for women!

VIAGRENE

Clearly intended to ride the wave of hype surrounding Viagra, this purportedly sex-enhancing carbonated drink is produced and bottled in Sweden and marketed by Eurofood-Link. The drink, blue in color, is being sold in Finland and Sweden. Pfizer, the maker of Viagra, has blocked the sale of Viagrene in Britain, accusing the manufacturer of violating its trademark. The drink's label declares that it is "the real drink for important moments" and has a design that Pfizer believes is similar to its pill design. A temporary ban on the sale of the drink in Britain has been issued until a full hearing can be held. The drink contains damiana, schizendra, mate, guarana, tropical fruits, acids, sugar, preservatives, coloring, water, and carbonation. Because it contains caffeine, it is not recommended for children, pregnant women, or those sensitive to caffeine. The soft drink is currently not available in the United States.

5 NATURE'S HELPING HAND

HERBAL ALTERNATIVES

For centuries, people throughout the world have used a wide variety of herbs to treat erectile dysfunction and low libido and to enhance the overall enjoyment of the sexual experience. Today's herbal practitioners see ED as a symptom that challenges us to make lifestyle changes; rather than treating the symptom in isolation, herbalists realize that sexual dysfunction may have complicated roots, each of which needs to be addressed to restore health. While pharmaceutical solutions may act quickly, if the underlying causes of ED remain, one becomes dependent on the drugs to function sexually. One advantage of most herbal alternatives is their gentle balancing nature. Herbs may work in a more leisurely fashion, but this gives us the time to absorb the changes they support. Regardless of whether one's ED stems from the stresses of modern life or from physiological disorders, herbs can certainly help replenish vitality and reduce tension, restoring the balance between mind and body that is so important for a positive sexual experience.

Some physicians even recommend *combining* Viagra with herbal remedies. The goal of this approach is to bring about immediate relief of ED symptoms through the use of Viagra, while allowing the herbs to slowly go to work on healing the underlying problem so that the Viagra can eventually be discontinued. This is a controversial and potentially risky practice, and it should only be undertaken under the guidance of a qualified physician.

Even when using solely herbal products, always take responsibility for your own health, because the market is only loosely regulated by the FDA. Herbal medicines can be powerful, and while most do not have dangerous side effects, some are toxic, especially in large quantities. Do not assume that doubling the recommended dosage will yield better or faster results; herbal remedies must be taken in moderation and with patience. In addition, be sure to purchase herbal supplements from a reliable supplier since good results depend on reliable products. It is always wise to consult an experienced herbalist, naturopath, or physician with herbal knowledge before embarking on an herbal regimen to be certain that a particular herb will not have an adverse effect if combined with other prescription drugs or health conditions.

This chapter covers a variety of herbs that have been used over the years with varying degrees of success to support a healthy sexual life. Certain botanicals are only beginning to be investigated as potential treatments for impotency and thus information about specific dosages and results is often limited. When available, scientific studies to support traditional uses are cited.

BLACK CUMIN SEED

Nicknamed the "blessed seed," this plant's botanical name is *Nigella sativa.* For thousands of years, black cumin has been used in the Middle East, Africa, and South Asia as a remedy for allergies, inflammation, and menstruation problems. It boosts morale and curbs depression and has also been used as a guard against bronchitis, asthma, neurodermatitis, poor digestion, and impotency. In the Hadith, a Muslim religious text, the prophet Muhammad said that black cumin oil "cures all illnesses except death." A small bottle of black cumin oil was found in the tomb of the pharaoh Tutankhamen.

Black cumin is an aromatic spice that looks somewhat akin to sesame seed except for its black color. Aside from its active ingredient, crystalline nigellone, it contains fifteen amino acids, proteins, carbohydrates, fixed and volatile oils, alkaloids, saponin, and crude fiber. Also in black cumin are the minerals calcium, iron, sodium, and potassium. Many of the more than one hundred active components in this healing seed have not yet been identified.

In the West, herbalists have long used black cumin oil to treat flatulence, dysentery, stomach and lung diseases, and jaundice. A diuretic, the oil also acts to increase nursing mothers' milk supply. Recent advances in chemistry lend credence to folk uses of the oil. More than two hundred studies at international universities have shown results that support uses of black cumin oil that were recorded almost fourteen hundred years ago. This herb has been useful in the treatment of diabetes melitus; it also promotes regularity, improves digestion, and combats intestinal worms and parasites.

In 1986 Dr. Peter Schleicher, an immunologist in Munich, examined black cumin oil to find new therapies for chronic diseases. He found this oil to be an ideal candidate for the prevention and treatment of cancer. Dr. Schleicher also found that black cumin oil cured allergies for about 70 percent of his patients. As a result of Schleicher's research, several of his colleagues in Munich have conducted more studies, finding black cumin successful in enhancing the immune system, as a bioregulator, as an anti-inflammatory, and as an aid for neurodermatitis. Studies have also shown that the herb is helpful for a variety of kidney and liver disorders as well as digestive problems. The antitumor effect of black cumin oil has also been scientifically established.

Unfortunately, research on impotency has thus far largely ignored the anecdotal evidence of black cumin's effectiveness. The herb has no known side effects and can be used safely. Black cumin can be taken in the form of herb or oil. If you should choose to take the oil, which is much more concentrated, exercise caution because many oil products are imported and may be adulterated or mixed with other oils. Some oils from the Middle East are extracted with heat and hexane, a petroleum by-product. Always choose a product that is labeled cold-pressed, solvent-free, and packed and sealed by machine. Try taking two capsules or one teaspoon of oil three times a day.

BOIS BANDE

In the West Indies, the bois bande tree is a well-known aphrodisiac. The bark of the tree is soaked in rum, then the rum is drunk for its sexually stimulating properties. Though there is strong anecdotal evidence of bois bande's effects, and even reports of dangerous priapisms resulting from its use, there have been no scientific studies to this point.

BROOM RAPE

Broom rape (*Cistanche salsa*) is a flowering plant found in northern China, Mongolia, and Siberia. It is used to stimulate sexual desire, as a tonic for the kidneys, and as a demulcent laxative. It is also said to lower blood pressure. The fleshy stems of the plant are used, rather than the flowers of the straightforward broom. The recommended daily dosage is 10 to 15 g.

CYPERUS

Used in China as an aphrodisiac and in Turkey as a stimulant, *Cyperus rotundus* is also known as tiririca. The roots and rhisomes treat a variety of disorders, including headaches, scorpion bites, wounds, sores, and fevers. It is an analgesic, antibacterial, astringent, anti-inflammatory, a tonic, and a stimulant.

DAMIANA

Damiana (*Turnera diffusa*) has been used as an aphrodisiac since ancient times, especially by the native people of Mexico. Related to the mint family, this small shrub with aromatic leaves is found in hot, humid climates throughout Mexico, Central and South America, in the West Indies, and in parts of Texas. Its leaves were originally used as medicine by native populations in several parts of Central America. Ancient Aztecs frequently used damiana leaves as a stimulant, second only to chocolate. In Mexico, children drink damiana as a tonic and popular beverage.

The Guayacure tribe in the Baja desert traditionally made a ceremonial cordial of damiana leaves. Legend has it that the Guayacure chief eventually banned its consumption because of its aphrodisiac powers. Today, the cordial is given to young grooms by mothers-in-law anxious to become grandmothers. In Mexico, allopathic physicians use damiana to treat ED, exhaustion, and bladder disorders. It is also used for inflammation of the testicles and involuntary emissions. Some Mexican doctors even employ it as a brain tonic.

From 1888 to 1947, damiana leaf and elixir were listed in the National Formulary of the United States. Although the complex chemical actions of the herb have not been identified completely, it has been used for more than a hundred years in Western societies to improve sexual function in both men and women. Some of the plant's constituents include alkaloids, bitter, tannins, resin, pinene, and many other parts of the essential oil. The alkaloids may have a testosteronelike action, which may explain damiana's strong effects on the sexual organs. It may strengthen the male sexual system as a whole. The herb also acts as an antidepressant, a tonic, and a mild laxative. In Germany, the leaves are used to treat mental and nervous disorders and as a tonic for the hormonal and central nervous systems. Damiana is known in Holland for enhancing sexuality and for its overall positive effect on the reproductive organs.

The leaves and stems of the plant are used. They are gathered during flowering and then dried. This herb can be prepared in several ways. To make a tea, pour a cup of boiling water over two tablespoons of dried leaves. Steep for ten to fifteen minutes and drink three cups a day. You may wish to add sweetener or mint for additional flavoring, and the tea may be taken hot or iced. If you wish to make a cordial, let it sit long enough—the longer it sits, the better the taste. One quick recipe from Diana DeLuca's *Botanica Erotica: Arousing Body, Mind, and Spirit* is to take one cup of commercially prepared vanilla extract, two tablespoons of damiana leaves, and one tablespoon of sweetener. Let the mixture sit for a week before straining through a cheesecloth. Tablets or capsules may be taken in the amount of 400 to 800 mg three times per day, but the herb is generally more effective when combined with complementary herbs. Some of these include oats (for nerves) and kola or skullcap.

Dodder

Dodder has some charming folk names: beggarweed, hellweed, strangle tare, scaldweed, and devil's guts. Many of these names come from its poor reputation among farmers, as it gives bean crops a scalded appearance and sometimes strangles other plants in its threads. The seeds grow into thready stems that climb adjoining plants and put forth small vesicles that attach themselves to the stem or bark of the other plants. Dodder eventually lives completely on the sap of its unwilling host plant. A true parasite, it has no leaves and has globular heads of waxlike flowers.

The variety effective for ED and for premature ejaculation, *Cuscuta japonica*, originates in China and Japan. In his seventeenth-century text, Nicolas Culpepper recommended the herb for melancholy diseases, many diseases of the head and brain, and also for trembling of the heart, fainting, and swooning. Worldwide, dodder seeds are currently used for a variety of medical purposes. It is most well known as a tonic for kidneys; a nutrient for bones, sinew, and cartilage; and a tonic for the liver. In some cases, treatment with dodder improves vision.

Historically, the threads were boiled in water with ginger and allspice and used for urinary complaints and for kidney, spleen, and liver diseases because of its laxative and hepatic action. It has also been used to treat jaundice as well as sciatic and scorbutic complaints.

GINKGO BILOBA

If Viagra is considered a wonder drug by many, then ginkgo biloba is equally esteemed by those in the alternative medicine community. Students and the elderly take it to improve their memories, depressed persons take it to increase their energy, and ginkgo biloba also provides an effective treatment for ED. It aids circulation and gets the blood flowing to the right spots. For example, in one German study, male patients who took 60 mg of ginkgo extract daily experienced better blood flow to the penis within six to eight weeks. At the end of the eighteen-month study, this herb had helped half the men regain normal sexual potency. In fact, more than two hundred and fifty pharmacological and university studies have been published about ginkgo in the last twenty years, most employing an extract of the dried leaves called EGb761.

Ginkgo, a deciduous tree, has been cultivated in East Asia for hundreds of years. The tree was introduced to a garden in Philadelphia in 1784. Mature ginkgoes can grow to more than a hundred feet in height, and individual trees may live as long as one thousand years. Female trees only bear seeds when quite old, so a tree planted by one person might not be mature for two generations. One of its colloquial names, Kung-sun-shu, means "grandfather and grandson tree."

Ginkgo seeds and leaves are widely used in clinical practice in both China and Europe. The dried, processed seed, with its seed coat and pulp removed, is used for asthma, coughs, bronchitis, tuberculosis, frequent urination, and other disorders. Its seeds are somewhat sweet, but also bitter, astringent, and potentially toxic. Seeds are used to treat asthma and to improve vital energy.

The somewhat bitter leaves promote blood circulation, stop pain, benefit the brain, and are useful for the lungs. They are also used for arteriosclerosis, angina pectoris, and dysentery. Sometimes an infusion of boiled leaves can relieve chilblains. In Europe, ginkgo leaf extract is prescribed for heart disease, ringing in the ears, dementia, short-term memory improvement, and vertigo.

A recent study, performed at the University of California, San Francisco, looked at the long-term safety and efficacy of ginkgo biloba extract (GBE) for treating antidepressant-induced sexual dysfunction. Dr. Alan Jay Cohen notes the ability of ginkgo biloba extract to reverse antidepressant-induced sexual dysfunction in three patients studied for six to eight weeks. Each man was started on a course of GBE of 60 mg twice a day. Doses were then raised to 120 mg, twice a day for four weeks, and later to 240 mg per day. The highest dose effectively reversed sexual dysfunction in all three patients. These men had a single episode of nonpsychotic major depression and no other medical or substance abuse problems. The only adverse reactions, which did not impede treatment, were some gastrointestinal complaints and a bit of lightheadedness.

For most people, ginkgo has a safe and positive effect on sexual functioning if 50 mg is taken three times a day. However, ginkgo does have possible contraindications and moderation is key. This is a case in which too much of a good thing can be dangerous. The fresh fruit pulp and the processed seeds of ginkgo are potentially poisonous. In large doses, more than ten seeds, they can have a toxic or even fatal effect. Side effects may include skin disorders or mucous membrane irritations. Also, eating the fresh seeds can cause stomachache, nausea, diarrhea, difficulty breathing, or shock. The fresh fruits of the tree may cause contact dermatitis, like poison ivy rash, and should be handled with rubber gloves.

GINSENG

For centuries, ginseng has been known as a stimulant and a panacea for a variety of ailments. It is certainly considered by many, especially in Asia, to be an aphrodisiac, although few scientific studies have supported this claim. Considered a restorative, not a curative, *Panax ginseng* is a fascinating plant, grown in a variety of countries. For the purposes of this book, only Asian ginseng, which is supposedly the most effective for sexual dysfunction, will be addressed.

Asian ginseng is grown in the mountains of eastern Asia and in Korea and Japan. It grows both in the wild (now extremely rare) and is cultivated. The Chinese *Panax ginseng* is perhaps the most effective in increasing men's vital energy, although Siberian ginseng (actually not ginseng at all but *Eleutherococcus senticosus*) is also a restorative. *Panax* comes from the Greek *pan-axos*, meaning all-curing, from the same root as the word *panacea*.

Ginseng is an erect plant that grows from eight to fifteen inches high and bears three leaves at its summit. Taking about six years to mature, the plant must be grown in rich, moist soil and watered frequently. Ginseng has a thick, spindle-shaped root, often branched. It is this branched root, especially if it resembles the shape of a human phallus, which finds particular favor with the Chinese, many of whom consume this root on a daily basis.

The Chinese have used this plant for thousands of years, although reports about just how long vary. Early Chinese believed that the best results were obtained when the root was dug up at midnight during a full moon. A rich mythology exists about ginseng, especially in China. One story about the discovery of this helpful root involves an entire village, Shantang, which was disturbed nightly by strange howling noises. The villagers gathered together and marched to investigate its sources. Finding a large bush, they dug it up and found a massive man-shaped root underneath, yelling to gain their attention. They named this root "spirit of the earth."

Many Asians cook the root with chicken to make a soup, believed to be a general restorative, and the more wealthy Chinese often use the root every day, chewing it, using its powder in hot tea, or ingesting it in extract form. In particular, Korean, Japanese, and Chinese men believe that ginseng enhances sex. An ancient medical manuscript of India, the Atherva Veda, notes that ginseng "bestows on men both young and old the power of a bull."

A fourth-century Chinese *materia medica* lists several exotic ginseng recipes to increase sexual appetites. A Chinese emperor, Shen-Nung, who believed in alchemy and sex for rejuvenation, recorded that he felt both warmth and sexual stirrings after chewing ginseng root. The *Pharmacopoeia* of Shen-Nung recommends the root to repair the five viscera, harmonize energies, strengthen the soul, and allay fear, and promises that continuous use will prolong life.

Ginseng is rich in vitamins B_1 and B_2 and contains phosphorus, iron, aluminum, copper, manganese, cobalt, sulfur, and silica. It also contains a steroid nucleus, which may be the key in explaining ginseng's regulatory and curative properties. Besides being considered an aphrodisiac, ginseng is also noted as useful for a number of conditions, including aging problems, wounds, stress, depression, ulcers, diabetes, headaches, and fatigue.

Ginseng can be found as a dried root, or as a tincture, powder, or liquid extract. Try taking 100 mg of the extract one to three times per day. Ginseng can also be made into a tea, which should be sipped slowly. However, as is true with many over-the-counter supplements, grave differences in quality are noted within the substance. Recent consumer tests revealed a wide variation in the amounts of six ginsenosides in ten different brands of commercially available ginseng. Be sure to purchase the herb from a reputable supplier.

Several side effects have been noted from ginseng use: it can cause high blood pressure as well as abnormal bleeding in postmenopausal women. Researchers warn against using ginseng over extended periods. After taking the herb for three weeks, take a two-week break. Other side effects of high usage may include nervousness, sleeplessness, skin eruptions, or morning diarrhea.

Nevertheless, thousands of Asian men continue to believe in the restorative capacity of this phallic-shaped root. Dr. Andrew Weil tells of a Chinese man who advised him against "wasting" ginseng in his youth: "He said to save it for my old age and then see what it could do for me."

KAVA

Often called the "Pacific elixir," kava (*Piper methysticum*) originates in the South Pacific where it has been used for millennia by the native peoples of Melanesia, Polynesia, and Micronesia. This slow-growing shrub is found throughout these islands and favors their tropical climate. The traditional method of preparation consisted of having groups of people chew and spit kava root into a big bowl. Coconut milk was added to the masticated mass and the resulting liquid was strained and drunk. In addition to serving important social functions for native peoples, kava was also used medicinally to treat a variety of conditions, including problems of the female reproductive system, headaches, weakness, insomnia, respiratory illnesses, and nervousness.

While kava does not seem to have been used as a traditional indigenous remedy for erectile dysfunction, recent research confirms kava's effectiveness in reducing stress and anxiety and relieving bladder and sleep disorders. The medicinally active constituents of kava are kavalactones (also called kavapyrones), which have mood-altering effects. Thus this root may be of use in resolving sexual difficulties and low libido caused by overwork, anxiousness, and tension. However, rumors notwithstanding, there is no reason that kava would have any effect in cases of true ED.

Kava is now readily available in the United States and in western Europe as commercially prepared extracts. The recommended dose is 70 to 210 mg of kavalactones three times a day. Low to moderate doses are recommended for relaxation since higher doses promote sleep. Initial clinical studies of kava extract have shown the root to be safe if used in moderation, but overdoses can cause unpleasant side effects such as dry skin, shortness of breath, blood disorders, and liver damage. Kava should not be used by anyone with Parkinson's disease.

KOLA NUT

Kola nut (*Cola nitida*) contains caffeine and other substances such as theobromine and kolamin in its seeds, which may explain its stimulating properties and actions. Brazilians drink it in a popular beverage, and Jamaicans use it as an aphrodisiac.

MACA

This Peruvian herb, *Lepidium peruvianum Chacón,* is just beginning to gain a following in the United States, primarily over the Internet. Maca is used to treat a wide variety of hormone imbalances, much like *Panax ginseng.* Scientists believe that it increases fertility, and some users claim that it increases sexual vigor although studies have not yet confirmed this. Studies *have* confirmed that rats fed maca had significantly higher sperm production. Maca is a member of the cabbage, cauliflower, and broccoli family and currently comes in capsules or dried powder. It is a nutritional goldmine, full of amino acids, calcium, phosphorus, zinc, magnesium, iron, iodine, steroidal glycosides, and vitamins B_1, B_2, B_{12}, C, and E. The herb is nontoxic and thus in moderate amounts it may be safely used to stir the libido.

MINT

Mint comes in many varieties (*Mentha piperita, Mentha aquatica,* and *Mentha spicata*) and can be purchased dried or fresh. Growing your own in a pot or in the ground is simple and provides a steady source of the fresh herb. Hippocrates recommended mint as a "love-brew," and the Greeks forbade their soldiers to consume it for fear of diminishing their courage. The Roman apothecary Dioscorides thought that all mint species were equally efficacious for sexual intercourse. It is purported to have tonic and stimulating properties and to induce genital well-being.

MUIRA PUAMA

Grown in Brazil's Amazon and Orinoco basins, muira puama has traditionally been used as an effective treatment for impotency. A small tree, it grows in the forests and jungles of South America. The tree, which grows to sixteen feet in height, has white flowers with an intense smell somewhat like jasmine. Its nicknames include "potency wood" and "tree of virility." Muira puama is used throughout the world as an aphrodisiac and is also noted as a treatment for neuromuscular problems such as rheumatism as well as paralysis and beri-beri. It is said to prevent baldness and to be useful for self-reflection.

All parts of the plant have been used historically, but the bark and roots are employed most often for medicinal reasons. Muira puama has been long
used by indigenous peoples for a number of purposes;
it has been used as an accepted herbal medicine in
South America and Europe since the 1920s.

Many clinical studies have been done on its effects. In 1925 a published study showed its effectiveness for treating nervous system disorders and sexual
impotency. In 1930 French experiments noted the
plant's use for gastrointestinal and circulatory asthenia and impotency. Muira puama has long been used
in England and is listed in the *British Herbal Phar-*
macopoeia, a respected tome from the British Herbal
Medicine Association, which recommends it for both
dysentery and ED.

More recent research has concluded that muira
puama's active constituents are free long-chain fatty
acids, sterols, coumarin, alkaloids, and essentials oils.
A recent study of 262 male patients at the Institute of
Sexology in Paris, France, all experiencing lack of
sexual drive and the inability to attain or maintain
an erection, suggests the herb is indeed effective.
Within two weeks, 62 percent of the patients believed
that the extract of muira puama was responsible for
dramatic improvements and 51 percent felt it was
beneficial. A second study in France, conducted by
Dr. Jacques Waynberg at the same institute, addressed the positive psychological benefits of the herb
in one hundred men with male sexual asthenia.

Testor-Plus is an extract of muira puama that
has also been evaluated extensively. The use of
Testor-Plus alone was studied in one hundred ur-
ban European men over the age of eighteen who were

experiencing sexual difficulties. The dosage regimen consisted of six oral doses a day for ten-day periods. The men's conditions were evaluated on the first day, the fifteenth day, and the thirtieth day. Frequency of intercourse increased significantly for sixty-two couples. Thirty-two patients felt a stronger libido. Twelve men said morning erections were improved. The stability of erection during intercourse was reestablished in fifty-two out of the ninety-four cases in the study. The researchers concluded that Testor-Plus provided a safe and effective herbal alternative to drugs.

Muira puama can be taken in many ways. A tea is most effective for treating impotency. Native people chewed the bark or cooked it to make a tea. They boiled two to four tablespoons of the shaved wood in one pint of water. A couple would drink one cup of the strained liquid one to two hours before sex. The herb can also be smoked or simmered in brandy.

Muira puama does have some side effects, however. More than 70 percent of people experience chills running up and down the spine two hours after taking the raw herb in capsules. There can also be an allergic reaction to the resins. An allergy test can be performed by scratching the skin with a sterilized pin and applying a sample of the herb. Make the scratches one-half-inch long, not deep enough to draw blood. If the scratch causes an irritation within sixty minutes, avoid this herb.

NETTLE

The Latin name is *Urtica dioica*, coming from *uro*, which means "I burn." The leaves of the plant are covered with little hairs that sting when placed in contact with the skin. From ancient Greece to the present day, nettle has been documented as a nourishing tonic that strengthens all the systems of the body. Nettle has been used by traditional herbalists to treat coughs and tuberculosis, increase hair growth, and relieve arthritis. It also may be supportive in benign prostatic hyperplasia, hay fever, high blood pressure, congestive heart failure, PMS, scurvy (because of its abundant vitamin C), and gout; it may relieve symptoms of prostate enlargement, hence its connection with impotency. Nettle is a diuretic, so replacing potassium in the body is essential. It is sometimes used by Native American women to strengthen the fetus and ease childbirth.

Nettle is found growing in the wild in moist, nitrogen-rich soil in somewhat shady areas where it draws the minerals from the soil into its leaves. One study concluded that polysaccharides and lectins are probably the active constituents. Rich in iron and vitamin C, nettle leaf has been shown to be anti-inflammatory; it prevents the body from making inflammatory chemicals known as prostaglandins. The root of the plant has complicated effects on hormones and proteins that carry sex hormones (such as testosterone or estrogen), which may explain why it helps benign prostatic hyperplasia. The leaves of the young plant are sometimes used in a salad, or slightly cooked like tiny spinach leaves, and its tough fibers have been used in cloth.

Nettle may be taken in several ways. For benign prostatic hyperplasia, herbalists often recommend 240 mg per day in capsules or tablets. Saw palmetto or pygeum may be combined with nettle root for particularly favorable results. Nettle can also be made into a tea by steeping a handful of leaves overnight in a quart of boiled water; strain and drink one or two cups daily. Alternatively, the herb may be steeped in wine, refrigerated, and sweetened with maple syrup or another favorite sweetener if desired. Traditional herbalists recommend a tea combining nettle juice, plantain juice, and juniper berries to cure ulcers of the stomach and intestines.

Nettle should not be given to very young children, and older children and the elderly should take only small doses. For long-term medicinal use, it is appropriate to consult with a physician. Large doses may cause stomach irritation, burning skin, and urinary suppression. Also, when contact is made with the skin, fresh nettles may cause a rash. Some recommend drinking the juice of the flowers to cure the sting.

ROSEMARY

This wonderfully scented shrub (*Rosemarinus officinalis*) grows wild in Mediterranean climates. It is especially popular in the region and cuisine of Provence. Archeological digs reveal that branches of rosemary were placed in Egyptian sarcophagi. In the pre-Christian era, the plant was considered sacred and used frequently in religious and funerary rites. Rosemary was thought to assist and preserve love if used during nuptial ceremonies.

The herb is also used medicinally, producing an antispasmodic effect on the digestion and assisting in the draining of bile. Rosemary's beneficial action on the adrenal glands, which produce sex hormones, helps to explain its aphrodisiac properties.

SAFFRON

Saffron comes from purple crocuses, *Crocus sativus*, and is prized from Italy to China for its pungent flavor and exquisite color. Much of the food to which it is added is considered erotic in taste and in color. Saffron was used by the ancient Phoenicians as a love spice to flavor moon-shaped cakes eaten in honor of Ashtoreth, the goddess of fertility. It is also still used as a bridal spice and as a beautiful golden yellow dye for foods like saffron rice in Cuban cuisine. It is considered to make erogenous zones more sensitive and also to have a hormonelike effect.

Saffron is one of the most expensive herbs in the world, yet its taste is worth it. The painstaking process of picking and drying the flowers' stigmas makes it so expensive. The crocuses grown in Spain produce the best saffron; their stigmas are longer and contain higher levels of the pigments and oil that give the herb its distinctive color, flavor, and aroma. The peak production of the flowers lasts only a week to ten days in October and November; cultivation is primarily in Castille and in Aragon. Most of the peelers are women, who strip away the petals and pluck out the stigmas by hand. An experienced peeler can go through ten to twelve thousand flowers in one day. It requires 250,000 to 300,000 flowers to produce the twelve pounds of stigmas required for two pounds of saffron.

SAVORY

Like rosemary, savory *(Satureja hortensis)* is a Mediterranean plant. The Greeks and Romans considered it sacred, using it in fertility rites. Savory has always been considered a potent aphrodisiac and specifically an aid for men who have difficulty performing the sexual act. Savory is also recommended for overtiredness and depression. Try making a tea with 3 teaspoons of dried herb for one cup of water.

SAW PALMETTO

Saw palmetto (*Serenoa repens*) has long been considered an aphrodisiac by herbalists, and modern medicine now recognizes this herb as a powerful remedy for enlarged prostate glands. Some sexual dysfunction in males can be traced directly to the prostate gland. Saw palmetto is also of value in infections of the gastrourinary tract. It is currently being studied to treat hirsuitism (abnormal hair growth) and polycystic ovarian disease in women.

The saw palmetto tree, also called the dwarf palm, is a native of the area from South Carolina to Florida, growing to a height of three to nine feet. It has fan-shaped silver, blue, or green leaves. The drug is derived from the ripe berries, about the size of olives, which range from bright red to brown at harvest time. They are gathered from early fall through midwinter. Native Americans in the southeastern United States have used these berries for centuries as an important food source and for strength. They provided nutrition after a hot summer and were valued for their effects on the reproductive health of both men and women.

The berries contain a volatile oil, a fixed oil, steroidal saponins, and other elements that make them useful for relieving colds, asthma, and bronchitis as well as urinary and reproductive disorders. Saw palmetto inhibits an enzyme that converts one type of testosterone to another, which may be important in the development of an enlarged prostate.

During a recent three-year European trial with 309 men, saw palmetto was associated with an impressive increase in urinary flow rate and a 50 percent decrease in residual urine volume. In comparison, the prescription drug Proscar showed a much smaller decrease in symptom scores over the three years. Only 1.8 percent of the participants experienced any side effects from taking saw palmetto. Saw palmetto is approved by the German government as a treatment for benign prostate enlargement, as are nettle root extracts and pumpkin seeds. In the United States, over-the-counter drugs to treat this condition have been banned, although saw palmetto is still available as a nutritional supplement.

The berries can be taken in several ways. A saw palmetto herbal extract is available in capsules or tablets, which are rich in fatty acids, sterols, and esters. A powdered dried fruit can be used as a tea, which is weaker than the herbal extract. Liquid extracts are also available. To make a tea, take one-half to one teaspoon of berries and boil them in a cup of water; simmer on low for five minutes. Drink three cups a day. Alternatively, you can add 1 to 2 ml of saw palmetto tincture to another liquid three times a day. Sometimes the berries are combined with damiana and kola for reproductive system problems. If you decide to take saw palmetto berries for a prostate condition, do so only after a thorough examination and diagnosis by your physician. Although the herb has no significant side effects and is nontoxic, it is important to confirm that a prostate condition is indeed benign before self-medicating.

ST. JOHN'S WORT

The conventional treatments for clinical (major) depression provide a classic example of how a pharmaceutical approach to disease may not be the most appropriate one. Depression often leads to a lack of interest in sex, but ironically the most popular synthetic drugs used to treat depression can themselves cause ED, decreased sexual desire, delayed ejaculation, or inability to ejaculate. Studies have shown that about 30 percent of patients taking standard drugs for depression experience sexual difficulties as a side effect. When mild to moderate depression is the root problem of ED or low libido, St. John's wort (*Hypericum perforatum*) may offer a botanical answer.

An unassuming, low-growing plant with yellow flowers, St. John's wort has been the subject of intense media attention over the past few years. Multiple clinical trials support what folk herbalists have known for centuries: St. John's wort is remarkably effective in relieving depression and anxiety without significant side effects. In fact, in double-blind studies, participants taking a placebo experienced side effects more often than those taking the herb. (A potential side effect at extremely high dosages is increased sensitivity to the sun, but this effect is very rare.) Commercially prepared, standardized forms of St. John's wort are the most effective form to use; the recommended dosage is 300 mg of St. John's wort three times per day with meals. Be sure to purchase a product that offers capsule, tablet, or tincture standardized to contain 0.3 percent hypericin, the plant's active constituent.

Depression is a serious health condition and anyone contemplating St. John's wort as an alternative to prescription antidepressants should consult their physician before discontinuing their medication. Combining St. John's wort with a synthetic antidepressant should only be done under a physician's supervision because scientists are not yet sure how the botanical medicine interacts with certain classes of drugs.

THYME

Perhaps those who suffer from erectile dysfunction should consider moving to a Mediterranean region and eating freely of its herbs. Thyme (*Thymus vulgaris*) is yet another herb that grows wild all over this sunny region; it is also cultivated in the south of France. Thyme has medicinal properties as a stimulant and is especially useful for sexual dysfunction caused by exhaustion or overtiredness.

TRIBULUS TERRESTRIS

Bulgarian athletes traditionally use *Tribulus terrestris* before important competitions, and in Europe it apparently has a long folk history of being used for hormone insufficiency. The herb, also known as caltrop or puncture vine, grows in moderate climates, primarily in the Indian subcontinent and Africa, and has been used as a diuretic, cooking tonic, and to combat renal disorder. *Tribulus terrestris* has also been used as an aphrodisiac and as a remedy for ED. The plant is touted for its ability to stimulate natural production of testosterone, which if true would make it useful for boosting low libido levels but useless in treating ED. Too little is known in the West about *Tribulus terrestris* to recommend long-term dosing. If you decide to experiment with this herb, take modest amounts, four weeks on followed by one week off.

VALERIAN

Herbalists have used valerian (*Valeriana officinalis*) for centuries as a safe and effective relaxant. Hildegard von Bingen, a twelfth-century herbalist, abbess, and mystic, recommended the herb as a cure for pleurisy or gicht, and valerian was one of the most popular herbs of the sixteenth century. Many over-the-counter medications sold in Europe as remedies for tension continue to include valerian. Scientists believe that the rhizomes and roots of this strongly scented plant contain sedative iridoids called valepotriates, which may be responsible for the herb's actions.

Because one's mental and emotional states are so connected to sexuality, anxiety and tension can have profound and negative effects on sexual functioning and desire. Valerian, although not specifically indicated for erectile dysfunction, may be of use if ED stems from a highly stressful professional or personal life. Valerian may also be of assistance if insomnia and exhaustion cause such disruption during the waking hours that a heathy sexual life seems impossible to achieve. Under the calming influence of the herb, sexual difficulties may gradually fade and be replaced with stronger and healthier sexual response.

Valerian is safe for long-term use and is not addictive. Dosage will depend on personal response to the herb. Valerian's strong smell makes it less enticing as a tea, and thus capsules, tablets, or tinctures will probably be preferred. Start off with perhaps a quarter of a teaspoon of the tincture or one capsule three times daily. If you do not feel a relaxing effect, gradually increase the amount of valerian taken until you find the dosage that works for you. The right dose should leave you feeling calmer but not groggy. Those taking valerian to relieve stress in an effort to improve sex drive will want to take more moderate doses than those taking the herb for insomnia. In rare cases valerian increases nervousness; if this happens to you, discontinue use of the herb.

VERBENA

Of the two types of verbena, lemon and officinal, the latter is the aphrodisiac. The Greeks considered it sacred to Aphrodite, goddess of love. The Romans considered it a good omen for peacemaking. If a messenger carried a verbena plant, it was taken as a sign of willingness to make peace.

An herbal tea can be prepared with verbena flowers, or verbena may be macerated for several days in a good quality wine. This is reputed to stimulate and augment the reactions of the body and to facilitate better circulation of the blood to the genitals.

YOHIMBE

Yohimbe is the only botanical to boast FDA approval as a remedy for ED. Ironically, in spite of this unusual government approval for an herb, U.S. research on yohimbe's effects on human males is still in its infancy, and the herb is also classified as an "unsafe herb" because it can cause serious side effects. The active substance is yohimbine, an alkaloid in the bark of the tree of the same name *(Pausinystalia johimbe)*, a native plant of tropical West Africa. The inner shavings of the bark act as a stimulant and aphrodisiac. The tree, which grows predominantly in Gabon, Nigeria, and the Cameroons, grows from twenty to fifty feet high, and has leaves from three to five inches in length. The seeds are winged.

Yohimbe is traditionally used by many Bantu-speaking tribes in a matrimony sacrament. It is used in mating rituals that have been known to last for up to ten or fifteen days. It has been used for more than seventy years as a treatment for both male and female sexual difficulties. Although yohimbe enjoys a reputation as an aphrodisiac among traditional practitioners, modern scientists have not been able to prove any effects on sexual drive in humans. The herb has been shown to increase sexual arousal and performance in male rats, but the effect in human males is yet unsubstantiated.

Yet, some statistics point to its usefulness as one herbal tool to treat impotency. One study from Rhode Island showed that yohimbe increases blood flow to the penis. In clinical trials, the active ingredient in the herb was tested on men impotent for less than two years. An improvement rate of 81 percent was reported for those who took a moderate dosage of the active ingredient for one month. More than 60 percent of the men who had experienced only partial erections and had failed at normal intercourse at least 50 percent of the time experienced fuller, longer-lasting erections and overall improved sexual function.

Earlier studies reported 70 to 85 percent "good to excellent" results with impotent patients. In the 1980s, a highly regulated landmark Canadian study showed that the active ingredient in the herb could be a significant aid for restoring potency in impotent diabetic and heart patients. This widely reported study reported a success rate for serious impotency cases of 44 percent.

In 1994, in Italy, a clinical study looked at impotent patients for eight weeks. Half received active tablets of yohimbe, half received placebos. The yohimbe group showed a 71 percent positive recovery rate; the placebo group showed a 22 percent recovery. When the placebo group was given the yohimbe tablets, their success rate climbed to 74 percent.

In a 1994 double-blind study, eighty-two men with erectile dysfunction and a high incidence of diabetes and vascular disease underwent a thorough evaluation. After one month of treatment with a maximum of 42 mg oral yohimbine hydrochloride daily, 14 percent of the men experienced full restoration of sustained erections. Twenty percent reported a partial response, and 65 percent reported no improvement. Only three men reported a positive effect from the placebo group.

Yohimbe can be taken in capsule or liquid forms, and requires a doctor's prescription. A standard dose is 15 to 20 mg per day, but higher doses, up to 42 mg, may sometimes be necessary. The effects of the herb take two to three weeks to manifest themselves. You may see yohimbe in health food stores in bark or extract form, but some of these may or may not have yohimbine in them. The pure yohimbine hydrochloride that seems to be the most effective in increasing libido and increasing blood flow to the penis must be obtained by prescription.

If you can find a reliable source for the raw herb, you can try preparing a tea or powder. To make a tea, bring two cups of water per person to a boil, adding one ounce of yohimbe to the boiling water, and boiling for less than four minutes. Then simmer the brew for twenty minutes longer. Strain the liquid and sip slowly about an hour before you desire its effects. To prepare a concentrated powder, soak one ounce of the bark shavings in ethyl alcohol, or any alcohol such as gin or vodka, for a full eight hours. Strain the shavings, and let the alcohol evaporate, which you may do in an oven set on the lowest heat. The residue will be predominantly yohimbine hydrochloride and can be snuffed or placed under the tongue. This preparation works more quickly than the tea.

Unfortunately, yohimbe's effectiveness is tempered by some significant side effects. It acts as both a central nervous system stimulant and as a mild hallucinogen. Thus, it is not recommended for men with mental disorders. Yohimbe may induce anxiety, panic attacks, and hallucinations in some people. Other side effects may include heightened blood pressure and heart rate, flushed skin, dizziness, and headache. An overdose can cause more serious problems: paralysis, fatigue, stomach disorders, and even death.

6 A Rose by Any Other Name

Traditional Aphrodisiacs

Somehow food and passion share a primal link. Eating in a more seductive way can only add spice to your sex life, whether or not you are also taking an herbal tincture or a vitamin supplement. Many of these aphrodisiacs have been known throughout the world for centuries, yet little concrete evidence exists for their effectiveness in increasing sexual prowess. They seldom do more than symbolize male potency, but some may contain male hormonal substances or vitamins, and others may enhance the mood of the evening or morning. In many cases, most aphrodisiacs are relatively harmless substances, especially in the case of vegetables and spices that you probably already have in your home kitchen. Animal substances, some from endangered or immature species, are another category altogether and will be discussed only briefly.

A look at Dr. William Hammond's *Sexual Impotence in the Male*, published in 1883, gives a different perspective than our modern one. Dr. Hammond believed that no such thing as an aphrodisiac or "special restorer of virility" was known to medical science. But he did believe there were agents that had an indirect, sometimes powerful influence in "giving tone" to the sexual organs or in alleviating conditions that caused ED. He assigned these agents to two categories: external and ingested.

Under external remedies, the first and highest recommended was electricity. Electricity (still used today in slightly different form) was used in three forms—Galvanism, Faradism, and Franklinism. Currents were applied to the spine, the perineum, the testicles, and the penis. Other external methods included massage, percussion, urtication, and flagellation. (The latter was applied to the buttocks.) The author denied any personal experience with any of these. Dr. Hammond defined urtication as flagellation performed with nettles.

Under the category of internal remedies, the author believed that in some cases the loss of sexual power was entirely mental and thus could be cured by whatever restored the confidence of the patient. Even an inert substance could cause a powerful response if the patient believed in the cure. Hammond went on to recommend certain medicines to improve the tone of the sexual organs as well as act on the nervous system as a whole. At the top of this list was phosphorus in the form of phosphides of zinc. He recommended giving a tenth of a grain three times a day in pill form, in solution, in oil, or in pure form. This needed to be taken for several weeks to produce any permanent effect. He also noted ointments containing phosphorus to apply to the penis and scrotum but added they were not terribly effective.

Other substances Hammond discussed were dilute hypophosphorus acid, a "pleasant-tasting" substance that decomposed quickly in the stomach. Dilute phosphoric acid, though not as powerful as the others, was also considered useful. Nux vomica and strychnia were also considered valuable "in the treatment of impotence coming from excess." Finally, Hammond noted the use of cod liver oil, which he employed often in his treatment of impotency.

Not all practitioners consider such methods antiquated. Because the mind may well be our most important sexual organ, stimulating the senses in their entirety cannot fail to be beneficial on some level. Several aphrodisiacs once in use are still reportedly quite effective. For example, several vegetables, both common and exotic, have gained a lengthy reputation for their supposed powers in the sexual arena. While sexual difficulties will probably not disappear after munching a stalk of celery, it certainly can't hurt to supplement natural remedies with some good food (you will want to avoid the rhino horn!). Why not plan a relaxing and romantic evening that begins with a carefully prepared meal and see what happens?

ALCOHOL

The use of alcohol to stimulate sexual vigor is of ancient origins. In *MacBeth*, act 2, scene 3, the porter says that "it provokes and it unprovokes; it provokes the desire, but it takes away the performance." Just how is it that alcohol builds desire but often squelches the follow-through action?

Wine, beer, and absinthe are all especially connected to the sexual drive and desires. Wine and hard alcohol remove inhibitions when drunk in small quantities. In very small quantities, alcohol can calm anxiety and induce exhilaration in those normally introverted. A shy person can gain a bit more courage. But when alcohol is taken in large doses, it can induce erectile dysfunction, or what the British call "brewer's droop." Being sick or sleepy certainly is not conducive to a romantic evening.

Wine is considered to be of divine origin and has always been praised as an aphrodisiac. The biblical Lot was made drunk by his daughters so he could recover his lost ardor. Bubbles from the seventeenth-century product of Champagne gave inspiration to lovers at that time. Casanova made his many conquests drink champagne. Madame de Pompadour, famous for her frigidity, stimulated her libido by drinking champagne after taking a nettle bath. And Louis XV's lovers knew how to seduce their royal lover: by serving him champagne.

Red burgundy wine, mixed with ginger, cinnamon, cloves, vanilla, and sugar, was known as Hippocrates' aphrodisiac and was heartily recommended by François Rabelais in *Gargantua and Pantagruel*. Another drink, *aqua mirabilis*, was used in the seventeenth century as both a strengthening tonic and as an aphrodisiac. Prepared by steeping finely ground cinnamon, galingale root, ginger, nutmeg, rosemary, and thyme in claret for one week, it

was then strained. One quarter bottle a day was considered a suitable dose.

Sometimes wine is the base to which one can
add some spices, such as vanilla and cardamom. Herbalist Diana De Luca also recommends adding flower
petals, leaves, and fresh fruit to white wines; roots,
spices, bark, and dried fruits to hearty red wines.

Beer is not considered an aphrodisiac, perhaps
because it often makes one feel bloated rather than
sexy. But in some countries stout is seen as an aphrodisiac. Two traditional remedies to stir the libido
have been combined in a new form. Oyster stout (see
Oysters, below), a recently concocted brew by
Murphy's of Ireland, contains extracts of oysters from
Ireland's west coast.

Absinthe, another alcoholic substance, is reputed to be quite potent as an aphrodisiac. It was
used extensively at the end of the last century by many
Europeans, especially French, and was popular with
artists and intellectuals. The primary force behind
an absinthe cult was the poet Paul Verlaine. Absinthe
was also used frequently by Charles Baudelaire and
Vincent van Gogh, who believed it stimulated creativity. Scholars believe some of van Gogh's highly col-
ored paintings may have been prompted by absinthe-
induced hallucinations. Pablo Picasso sculpted a glass
of absinthe in 1914, the year before it was prohibited
in many countries.

Absinthe is primarily an extract of wormwood,
a plant rich in quite toxic compounds, such as the
essential oils thujone and thujol. Frequent use of
thujone, considered a convulsant, can result in blind-
ness, cramps, and nerve injuries. Thujone occurs in

a variety of plants, including tansy and sage. Wormwood and Roman wormwood are the primary sources
of thujone in absinthe.

Absinthe was prohibited in France in 1915 and
is still banned in most European countries because
of its toxicity. Absinthe, made with wormwood, is still
available in Spain, Denmark, and Portugal. Other
drinks related to this strong stuff are pernod (absinthe
without the wormwood), vermouth, chartreuse, and
Benedictine, which all contain small amounts of
thujone.

ARTICHOKES

The artichoke is the immature flower bud of a perennial thistle. The sweet, tender heart is what we're all
after. One of the oldest foods known to humans, artichokes flourished in the Mediterranean region and in
the Canary Islands centuries ago. The ancient Greeks
and Romans swore by its arousing powers. It was the
most expensive vegetable of ancient Rome, and, by
the sixteenth century, a favorite food of nobility.

Some fifty varieties of the true artichoke, *Cynara
scolymus*, are known worldwide. Although most artichokes were once imported from France, they are now
grown in coastal California and are generally available year-round. It is the official vegetable of Monterey
County in California, an area distinguished for its fine,
often organic produce.

When cooking this green vegetable, it is important that you steam or boil in stainless steel, enam-
eled, or glass pots, because to do otherwise discolors
the chokes and imparts an off-flavor. Artichokes are

excellent for dieters. A twelve-ounce artichoke (with no butter or Bernaise sauce!) is only twenty-five calories, and it contains lots of vitamin C and no fat.

ASPARAGUS

Already its shape gives you a clue to its power. Cultivated early on by the Greeks, it belongs to the lily family. One Arab source indicates that asparagus should be boiled in water, then briefly fried in fat and sprinkled with condiments to best provide an aphrodisiac effect. One caution is necessary. According to a certain Quensel (1809), asparagus turns men on but turns women off. This could certainly ruin what appears to be a wonderful night's meal.

CARDAMOM

Cardamom is frequently used in Indian and Arab recipes. It is especially good in rice pudding and with some couscous main dishes. In a traditional Indian remedy for ED and premature ejaculation, powdered cardamom seeds are boiled with milk and taken with honey before bedtime. Taken in excess, however, the same concoction could also increase impotency. Cardamom is mentioned frequently in the Kama Sutra, especially used in alcohol and in appetizers.

CELERY

Again, this vegetable's shape has a lot in its favor. Celery, rich in vitamins A and C, has long been used as an aphrodisiac. The stalks can be eaten raw but can also be boiled or braised. The root is best eaten peeled, julienned, or blanched. The seeds, crushed and added to a spicy bread or an oil-vinegar salad dressing, apparently work especially well as a sexual aid. Celery is low-calorie, fiber rich, and helps clean your teeth.

The Romans dedicated celery to their god Pluto, the god of sex and the king of the underworld. In the Middle Ages, some believed that celery could act even at a distance. If its stalks were placed under a pregnant woman's bed without her knowing, and if the first name she pronounced upon waking was a boy's name, she would, indeed, give birth to a boy. Researchers believe celery causes humans to excrete the male hormone androsterone through perspiration.

CLOVES

These dried flower buds have been considered an aphrodisiac in China since the third century B.C. In Europe, they also acquired some fame in this regard. A Swedish herbalist, Anders Mansson Rydaholm, wrote in 1642 that "if a man loses his ability, he should stay sober and drink milk spiced with 5 grammes of cloves. This will fortify him and make him desire his wife." The main ingredient of cloves and their oil is eugenol, earlier used as a dental analgesic.

FENNEL

Fennel is a perennial plant that grows well in vegetable gardens and flower borders. It is attractive and smells fresh, somewhat like anise. The Greeks regarded fennel as a potent sexual aid. During Dionysian festivals, crowns of fennel leaves were worn and its leaves and seeds were considered aphrodisiacs. According to the Kama Sutra, fresh fennel juice mixed with milk is an aphrodisiac. A traditional Hindu prescription for sexual vigor includes fennel juice, milk, honey, ghee, licorice, and sugar. Fennel soup is also popular as a sexual stimulant in Mediterranean regions.

GARLIC

What isn't garlic good for? It enhances every meal, settles a crampy stomach, and lends a certain *joie de vivre* to any occasion. Bah humbug to those who want to take it with no odor; the odor is one of its charms. Perhaps Sir John Harrington put it best in *The Englishman's Doctor* in 1609: "Garlic then have power to save from death / Bear with it though it maketh unsavory breath, / And scorn not garlic like some that think / It only maketh men wink and drink and stink."

The priestesses of the temples of Eros, Aphrodite, and Dionysus were all expert in making love potions. They attracted pilgrims from all corners of the empire to their sanctuaries. Garlic, washed in water and oil before consumption, was always a basic ingredient of their concoctions. Aristotle recommended garlic as a tonic, and Pliny the Elder taught that garlic, when pounded with fresh coriander and drunk with wine, was an aphrodisiac.

Chester Aaron, author of *Garlic Is Life*, tried this on his seventy-first birthday, but he doesn't tell us if it worked. After his twenty-year marriage ended, Aaron also ate garlic daily to distract him from thoughts about his broken marriage. This ritual apparently eliminated guilt and remorse.

Garlic belongs to the same genus as another reported aphrodisiac, the onion, and includes as many as seven hundred species. It has been used since early Egyptian times for many illnesses. It was also used as an aphrodisiac by Greeks, Romans, Chinese, and Japanese early on.

Garlic may even be used externally. Rubbing it on one's abdomen eases cramps, and David Berman, an emeritus professor of the University of Southern California Medical School, suggests crushing cloves of garlic, mixing them with lard, and rubbing them on an "unwilling" male member.

Most researchers believe the high sulfur content in garlic is the medicinally active agent. It is also an excellent source of biologically active selenium, which may normalize blood pressure and is a powerful antioxidant. Fresh garlic gives the maximum benefits, but because the fresh clove can irritate the digestive tract, it is best combined with oil and eaten on bread or with salad. Food seasoned with garlic becomes more appetizing, increases the appetite, smells great, and generally promotes a higher sense of well-being and joy. Where would we all be without it?

GINGER

Ginger provides pungent flavor in holiday cookies and in apple pie. But throughout Asia, and known as early as Pliny the Elder, ginger has also been used as a powerful aphrodisiac. Ginger ointments were used as stimulating massages for the abdomen. One pound of ointment of ginger, lilac, and pyrethrum (the plant, not the insecticide) is suggested for rubbing onto not only the abdomen, but also the scrotum and the anus. Some sources recommend its use both externally and internally. Indian literature suggests mixing ginger juice, honey, and half-boiled eggs, and taking this at night for a month as an ED remedy.

NUTMEG

Another holiday spice used in baking and in many soups, nutmeg also has a subtle aphrodisiac effect. It has been used by Hindus, Arabs, Greeks, and Romans. In Asia, it was especially prized as an aphrodisiac for women. An Indian recipe for increased sexual endurance calls for nutmeg mixed with honey and a half-boiled egg to be taken an hour before intercourse. Be aware, however, that high doses can produce quite severe hallucinogenic side effects.

OCTACOSANOL

Octacosanol, which has a reputation as an aphrodisiac, is a natural food supplement available in capsule form from health food stores. It contains wheat, wheat germ, and vegetable oils. The vitamins from these foods are thought to support healthy sexual appetites.

OYSTERS

As far back as the Roman Empire, oysters were considered an aphrodisiac. During the "Golden Century" in the Netherlands, the seventeenth century, they were the most frequently used aphrodisiac. Casanova is said to have eaten fifty oysters raw every morning while in the bath with whichever lady he fancied that day. A healthy food, oysters are low in fat and high in minerals, especially zinc, essential for a healthy reproductive system. They are usually eaten raw, are good with fresh lemon juice or Worcestershire sauce, and, of course, may be made into an excellent soup or stew. Some oysters, however, such as the Eastern oysters from the Chesapeake Bay of the eastern United States, are rapidly decreasing in numbers.

Sprouts

Sprouts—whether wheat, soy bean, oat, or alfalfa— are rich in essential vitamins, low in calories, and may add some zip to your diet. They can be sprinkled on salads and sandwiches or snacked on with other vegetables. The idea that consuming a food with symbolic import—in this case a sprouting seed representing regeneration—can act as an aphrodisiac is an ancient one. It may or may not be true, but your sandwich will certainly be tastier.

Truffles

Truffles have been known for centuries as an aphrodisiac. Most highly rated by the early Romans were those from Cyrene and Thrakia. Pliny suggests that truffles might be the result of a thunderbolt! Such energy is bound to be inspiring. In the late eighteenth century, the interest in the erotic powers of these un-derground fungi focused on the French variety. In *Physiologie du Gout*, published in 1825 by Anthelme Brillat-Savarin, the author devotes ten pages to truffles, noting, "Truffles are no perfect aphrodisiac, but in certain cases they can make women more yield-ing and men more amiable."

VANILLA

It's no surprise that sensual vanilla has long been con-sidered an aphrodisiac. Vanilla comes from a tree na-tive to the area around the Gulf of Mexico and north-ern South America. N.J. Berlin, in an 1849 message to the *Swedish pharmacopoedia*, noted that the sub-stance acted through both its odor and its taste.

Always use the natural product, not synthetic combinations, which are cheaper but not as potent nor as authentic. We bakers know this already. Va-nilla essence, extracted from the vanilla bean, may also be added to the bath, especially for lovers who want to bathe together. Vanilla can also be added to teas or to wine or juice. An old French recipe for a "love" wine combines Chablis, vanilla bean, cinna-mon chips, dried rhubarb, and ginseng. And you can't beat the fragrance of vanilla candles for setting a ro-mantic mood.

ANIMAL AND INSECT APHRODISIACS

Several supposed remedies for impotency involve the animal and insect world. Since ancient times, men have been convinced that virility can be obtained by eating other male animals, especially their genitals. The flesh of animals killed during the rutting period—particularly the sexual organs of bulls, donkeys, or deer—have been seen as possible cures for erectile dysfunction. As these are quite distasteful and involve endangered species on some counts, they will be treated lightly and briefly. None of these remedies is recommended!

ANIMAL GENITALIA

The penis and testicles of various animals are also often consumed in Asia for their aphrodisiac effects. Even today, after the kill, deer testicles are still carefully put aside. Organotherapy relies on extracts from animal testicles to supply the human body with testosterone. The use of deer genitals dates back to antiquity. Hippocrates recommends eating deer penis to resolve sexual difficulties. The Romans consumed genitalia from animals and birds: penises, wombs, and testes. The therapy is based on the belief that consumption of healthy animal organs might cure problems in the corresponding human organs.

Such practices may seem to belong to a lost era, but old beliefs persist. One Canadian company reportedly delivered 50,000 seal carcasses to China in 1994. The genitals of a seal fetched more than $100, while the pelt, meat, and oil went for $20. In a related report from 1998, DNA tests of what were called seal penises sold as aphrodisiacs in traditional Chinese medicine shops revealed that some were from domestic cattle, dogs, and protected seal species.

Such practices hurt more than consumers. David M. Lavigne of the University of Guelph in Ontario and his colleges identified twenty-one samples from shops in Toronto, Calgary, Vancouver, and San Francisco as well as others from shops in Bangkok and other Asian cities. Twelve specimens passed the test as legal seal products; eleven matched harp seal DNA, and another was probably a hooded seal. The other samples may have been Australian fur seal, which is illegal to hunt; domestic cattle or water buffalo; and African wild dog, a protected species. The science chief at the U. S. Fish and Wildlife Service's forensics lab in Oregon said that he could only remember finding three real seal penises in nine years of analyzing dozens of samples.

DEER ANTLERS

In Asian countries, powdered deer horn, gathered from reindeer, has long been considered an aphrodisiac; some recent scientific work has corroborated that the substance does contain male sex hormones although many experts doubt that ingesting such substances does anything to relieve erectile dysfunction. The Chinese pharmacopoeia includes tables of powdered deer horn, and shredded reindeer antlers are imported for aphrodisiac purposes from Canada, Finland, Norway, and Sweden to Japan. Some antlers are harvested responsibly when the animals shed them once a year. Unfortunately, others are not so scrupulous.

Fresh antlers are supposed to be the most powerful, but removal of live antlers from animals is forbidden in Scandinavia. In a sad related note, the Tibet red deer has long been listed as an endangered species, threatened with extinction because their velvety antlers are highly prized as an aphrodisiac. Once thought to be extinct, a herd of two hundred red deer was recently discovered in Tibet in the alpine meadows.

RHINO HORN

Powdered rhino horn is still prized in a few Asian and African countries as an aphrodisiac and remedy for headaches and food poisoning. Widespread poaching of rhinos has led to all five rhino species (three in Asia, two in Africa) being listed as endangered species. The use of rhino horns for medical purposes was declared illegal by the State Council of the People's Republic of China on May 29, 1993. However, some illegal trade may still continue.

SNAKE BLOOD

In parts of Eastern Asia, ingesting fresh snake blood from a poisonous snake is believed to boost the sexual drive. Cobras appear to be the favored species. A restaurant in Saigon supposedly offers a snake blood cocktail, cobra blood mixed with hard liquor; it also serves bat blood.

SPANISH FLY

Spanish fly is a golden-green iridescent beetle from which a chemical called cantharidin is extracted. This insect, with a body of fifteen to twenty-two millimeters long, is found on the leaves of ash trees in Mediterranean regions in the early summer. The Latin name of the beetle, *Lytta vesicatoria*, derives from the Greek: *lytta* means rage, *vesica* means blister.

Cantharidin is toxic to the kidneys and is an intense irritant to the genitourinary system. The poet Lucretius and twenty-five-year-old Prince de Conti, among others, died from its toxic effects. The mistress of Louis XIV, Madame de Montespan, gave her king "love powders" that contained cantharidin. The royal servants, in collusion with Madame de Montespan, added the concocted paste to the king's food to improve his sexual performance. Although he didn't die from ingesting the substance, Louis XIV experienced spells of giddiness.

7 LESS IS MORE

HOMEOPATHY AND
BACH FLOWER REMEDIES

Both homeopathy and the Bach flower system are based on the belief that curing the person, not the disease, is the goal of any health care treatment. Thus symptoms are useful signs that point us toward areas in need of change. Suppressing the symptom without addressing the cause is seen as shortsighted. Such an approach views ED as an imbalance that must be addressed holistically. When balance is restored to the entire person—emotionally, physically, and spiritually —a rejuvenated sexual life often follows. Because both healing modalities use minute dosages of natural materials, they are entirely safe and without any side effects. The choice of remedy is closely tied to an individual's particular case, so two men with ED may find success with two completely different remedies. Homeopathic remedies and Bach flower therapies work especially well in concert with sex therapy.

HOMEOPATHY: A GENTLE SOLUTION

German physician and chemist Samuel Hahnemann founded modern homeopathy at the beginning of the nineteenth century. Homeopathic medicines are prepared with substances from the animal, vegetable, and mineral kingdoms. Plants are harvested in their natural habitat by specialists and brought in their fresh form for laboratory conversion. Venoms, hormones, and organs of animals are used for extracts. Mineral salts and metals are treated in the laboratory. A preparation known as the mother tincture results from the maceration of plants and other base products in alcohol. This tincture is the initial source that will then be diluted into infinitesimal doses for the preparation of a given homeopathic medication.

How do homeopathic remedies work? Based on the ancient Law of Similars in which "like cures like," homeopathy works on the premise that a substance that causes symptoms when given in large amounts to a healthy individual will cure similar symptoms when given in highly diluted amounts to an ill individual. Some homeopaths explain that the remedies work by stimulating the body's natural defenses, which causes an individual to regain health.

Homeopathic medications come in the forms of granules, doses, globules, or drops. Drops are generally taken before meals with water. Granules and doses are placed under the tongue, where they melt. The remedies are labeled with the remedy name and a potency number (for example, 6c or 6x, or 30c or 30x). The higher the potency number, the more diluted the dosage but the more powerful the remedy.

Homeopathic medication should not be touched with the fingers because the medication's surface is active. It is meant to be poured directly into the mouth from the capsule in which it is contained. If you drop a pill, throw it out; do not return it to the bottle. Also be sure to store homeopathic remedies in their own tightly sealed bottles away from strong light or odors.

Mint should be avoided when taking any homeopathic treatment. Mint tea, mint-flavored chewing gum, and mint syrup should not be taken. A special mintfree toothpaste has been developed for people taking such treatments.

The following homeopathic remedies are safe for home use. If one remedy does not prove effective, feel free to try another. The process of finding the right remedy for a particular individual's case is often one of trial and error. The wrong remedy will not resolve the difficulty but it will not be harmful.

HOMEOPATHIC TREATMENTS FOR SEXUAL DISORDERS

Symptoms	Remedy
Inability to achieve erection, particularly after urethral or seminal discharges	Agnus castus
For small or fat men with strong sexual urges who cannot achieve an erection	Calcarea carbonica
For oversexed men who suffer from ED and experience involuntary loss of semen, diarrhea, or headaches	Cinchona

HOMEOPATHIC TREATMENTS FOR SEXUAL DISORDERS *(cont'd)*

Symptoms	*Remedy*
For men with intense sexual desires who cannot satisfy them and who ejaculate prematurely or involuntarily, particularly in the presence of women; for men who experience sexual difficulty after prolonged abstinence or excess	Conium maculatum
For shy or overanxious men who fear failure	Gelsemium
For ED accompanied by insomnia or overintellectualism; for psychiatric convalescents	Kalium phosphoricum
For young men with ED despite desire for sex, often big eaters and sedentary	Lycopodium clavatum
For all ED with psychological roots	Onosmodium
For premature ejaculation, often with oily skin or hair loss	Selenium
For the solitary man with ED	Sepia
For ED with sexual obsession; excessive masturbation; for backache following excessive intercourse	Staphysagnia

BACH FLOWER REMEDIES: WHEN EMOTIONS ARE THE KEY

These remedies were developed by Dr. Edward Bach, a physician from Mount Vernon, England, who lived from 1880 to 1936. He found thirty-eight flowers that are ideal for use in healing negative emotional states. In 1930 he gave up his practice to devote himself to finding plant essences that would restore vitality and enable the patient to assist in his own healing process. Subsequently, in 1978, twenty-four new flower remedies were discovered in the United States using Dr. Bach's theories.

The remedies are prepared from the flowers of wild plants, bushes, and trees; none of them is harmful or addictive. The mother tincture is prepared from the maceration of flowers in pure spring water that has been exposed to the sun for a few hours. The principle of the therapy is that the psychological aspect at the root of an illness is more important than the symptoms being experienced by the physical body. Bach believed that a state of sustained worry or fear depleted an individual's vitality. By taking the appropriate remedy over time, peace and harmony can be achieved and the body can heal itself.

Bach remedies are benign in action and produce no unpleasant reactions. More than one remedy may be taken at a time. Some herbalists recommend that two drops of each chosen remedy be put in a glass of water and sipped at intervals throughout the day. However, one may take four to seven drops of the remedy, placing the drops directly under one's tongue, three to four times a day. It is critical to keep the solution under the tongue for a few moments before swallowing the remedy. The medication will be more easily absorbed if you do so.

Following are the Bach flower remedies most appropriate for psychological conditions relating to impotency.

BACH FLOWER REMEDIES FOR SEXUAL DISORDERS

Indications	Remedy
Sexual inhibition	Basil
Internal conflict linked with trauma	Bleeding heart
Repulsed by earthiness of sex	Crab apple
Fear of loss of control	Cherry plum
Illness from subconscious conflicts	Fuchsia
Mental blocks of sexual origin, repression	Hibiscus
Feelings of guilt for wanting sex	Pine
Performance anxiety, perfectionist	Rock water
Fears linked to sexuality	Sticky monkey flower
Critical life changes, transitions	Walnut

8 GET THE LEAD OUT!

DIET AND LIFESTYLE CHANGES

Because erectile dysfunction generally occurs in middle age, a variety of factors related to diet, exercise, aging, and stress may come into play. Many of these factors can be improved dramatically with lifestyle changes. Heavy smokers and drinkers have a higher risk for ED than those who smoke or drink moderately, or not at all. People with high cholesterol levels may have more trouble maintaining erections than those with lower cholesterol levels. Men who are overweight and out of shape in general may have more difficulty. Certainly people whose primary relationship is not emotionally satisfying often have less satisfactory sexual relationships.

The good news is that ED is not inevitable and it certainly can be reversed. According to Masters and Johnson, approximately 25 to 30 percent of people in their sixties have successful intercourse at least once a week. After exploring the aspects of your lifestyle that may be contributing to ED, you can make specific changes to support your own healing. Rather than diagnosing the causes of ED yourself, however, you should begin by having a full physical with a doctor who can help you determine the basis of the ED. Then you will be in a position to evaluate what lifestyle changes best suit your particular needs.

ON THE COUCH

There are many theories about the emotional components inherent in some cases of ED. Familial, social, and intrapsychic factors may all contribute to ED. Our culture encourages a number of beliefs that may interfere with a healthy sexual life. Men burdened with performance anxiety, troublesome relationships with their mothers, religious beliefs that view sexual desire as sinful, or anger toward women are more likely to experience sexual difficulties. Men whose first sexual experience was traumatic and men who fear impregnating their partners may also find satisfying sex elusive.

Although the relationship between depression and ED is not entirely understood, it is clear that the two conditions are often linked. A recent study of 1,265 men took place at the Boston University School of Medicine in which researchers found that those suffering with depression were about twice as likely as other men to suffer from ED. The authors of the report have not established a causative relationship between the condition, but recommend that doctors screen patients with erectile dysfunction for depression. A number of herbs show promise for treating mild depression without the side effect of ED, which may offer men a solution (see chapter 5).

Stress can be as harmful to the body as depression, and the years between the ages of forty and sixty usher in new and not always welcome circumstances. While we may become more self-aware and have the opportunity to see our accomplishments in action, we also experience challenges and changes to daily life that can be alarming at times. The cycle of life may newly acquaint us with the deaths of relatives and peers, and various physical ailments or setbacks begin to plague us. We may notice a decline of youthful strength and energies. Our parents die; many of us divorce; our adult children leave or return to our homes; we retire or start new careers. We may have sleep disorders and develop aches and pains.

A plethora of studies have documented the deleterious effects of stress on the human body. Western culture, with its emphasis on speed and constant activity, puts us in a distinct danger zone for the physical and psychological ailments that accompany nonstop stress. A person's reaction to stressful events is physiological. Heart rate and blood pressure increase; breathing speeds up. Stress can have a cumulative effect, causing sleep disorders, low energy levels, and inability to concentrate as well as altering sexual desires and functioning. The body-mind connection can be so strong that anxiety may directly cause ED. Researchers at the Male Health Center in Dallas, Texas, found that fear of not being able to achieve an erection can actually cause ED. The body actually responded to this fear by shutting down the blood flow to the penis.

In today's fast-paced society, nearly all of us are more stressed-out and depressed than we would like to be. If you feel that your life is spiraling out of control, you would do well to consider what you can change. Sometimes when we feel pressed for time, we can regain a measure of control by making a conscious effort to slow down and create time for the things we find relaxing. Or perhaps we need to admit to ourselves that it is time to seek the assistance of a therapist who can help us resolve troubling personal issues.

Unfortunately, it is not always possible to avoid the people or situations that are causing stress in our lives. And in many cases eliminating one stressor usually introduces a new one into the picture; if we quit our jobs we may not have to deal with our bosses but we face new financial stressors. The best way to take control of our lives again is to remind ourselves that while we may not be able to change our surroundings, we can change our response to stress. Probably the most helpful change we can make is to make exercise, meditation or relaxation, and healthy eating our top priorities. The sections and the chapter that follow will offer more information about how changes in diet and exercise can relieve stress and even lift depression.

WHAT YOU DON'T KNOW CAN CAUSE ED

As discussed in chapter 2, ED may be caused by medications intended to cure some other condition. Some medications, including those for blood pressure and glaucoma as well as certain antidepressants, may cause

ED as a side effect. Lisinopril and atenolol, two drugs used to treat high blood pressure, appear to cause sexual dysfunction. Researchers treated ninety men between the ages of forty and forty-nine who had no prior history of sexual dysfunction. In the first month of treatment, patients taking either one of these drugs reported decreased sexual activity levels. Previous studies have corroborated this link. Because high blood pressure, depression, and glaucoma are serious conditions, however, you should not stop taking any medications that your doctor has prescribed to treat them. But don't suffer in embarrassed silence. Instead, speak with your health care provider about finding an alternative medication or decreasing your dosage under medical supervision to see if ED can be improved.

TOSS THAT BUTT!

Several other lifestyle issues can affect one's ability to have a satisfactory erection and follow-through. Studies show that smoking and chronic alcoholism have strong ties to this dysfunction. James Barada, M.D., the facilitator for the American Urological Association Erectile Dysfunction Treatment Guidelines Panel, recently said that the three greatest causes of ED are "smoking, smoking, smoking!" Studies in Massachusetts, California, and elsewhere have backed this claim. In addition, the risk factors for cardiovascular disease—smoking, elevated cholesterol, high blood pressure, physical inactivity, and overweightness—are all associated with erectile difficulties. A 1994 study by the New England Research Institute revealed that among men with heart disease and hypertension, cigarette smoking was related to a greater probability of complete ED. Another study, by the Centers for Disease Control and Prevention, found that among 4,462 Vietnam-era vets ranging in age from 31 to 49, 3.7 percent of current smokers were sexually dysfunctional as compared to 2.2 percent of the nonsmokers. Perhaps knowing that smoking may be at the root of ED may provide the motivation some men need to finally break the habit.

Cigarettes and cigars increase plaque formation and damage arteries. The key to resolving ED is to promote healthy circulation of blood. Recent clinical studies have shown that arteries can be opened up again by eating a vegetarian diet, refraining from smoking, and getting regular physical activity. Limiting intake of coffee, black tea, and alcohol may also help because caffeine constricts blood vessels and alcohol inhibits testosterone production.

EATING YOUR WAY TO BETTER SEX

A healthy diet includes a wide variety of foods in moderately sized proportions. Limit fat, cholesterol, sodium, alcohol, and sugars. Eat sparingly of red meat and highly processed foods. High-fiber, complex carbohydrates, and monounsaturated or polyunsaturated fats are especially beneficial. Lay low on packaged and canned foods; eat as much fresh and organic produce as possible.

Changing your diet dramatically will no doubt be difficult; the food we eat touches our emotional centers. We feel uncomfortable at first with dishes that we find strange. But the effort you put into overhauling your way of eating will repay you a thousandfold. If your ED is caused by high blood pressure medication, it's possible that diet changes may enable you to reduce or eliminate the medication causing the ED. Likewise, a healthy diet can help you reduce your weight or cholesterol level, both of which may have a significant impact on your sexual functioning. Making any or all of these alterations in your daily diet will likely add years to your life and life to your years. If nothing else, improving your diet will increase your sense of energy and well-being—both important elements for a healthy sex life. The suggestions that follow are meant to introduce the basics as they relate to ED; there are also many books available that provide guides to healthy eating.

One recent study found that men with high cholesterol are twice as likely to be sexually dysfunctional as men with normal or low cholesterol levels. In a study of 3,250 men between the ages of twenty-five and eighty-three, those with cholesterol higher than 240 mg/dl were twice as likely to have trouble achieving or maintaining an erection as those with cholesterol levels below 180 mg/dl. A high-fat diet that narrows arteries and blocks blood flow to the heart also narrows the arteries carrying blood to the penis. Sufficient blood must reach the penis to achieve an erection.

The benefits of red wine have been in the news a lot in recent years. The French drink it almost every day, sometimes at two meals, and survive quite nicely. Despite their fat-laden diets and alcohol consumption, the French are two and a half times less likely to die of coronary heart disease than Americans. According to a Johns Hopkins Adult Health Advisor bulletin, men should have two drinks a day at most—five ounces of wine or one can of beer, or a small drink of another liquor. In a research review released in March 1999, researchers found, based on a study of 28,160 men and women, that among men, a high consumption of spirits and beer increased the risk of cancer, yet wine in moderate amounts may offer protection against the possibility of lung cancer. Moderate alcohol consumption may also reduce risk of ischemic stroke (the most common sort of stroke), possibly by raising the "good" HDL cholesterol levels.

Moderation in alcohol consumption is the key to reaping potential benefits. Most doctors and other health experts stress that excessive alcohol consumption may lead to weight gain, liver disease, brain damage, and other serious disorders. The National Institute on Alcohol Abuse and Alcoholism found that prolonged alcohol use is associated with brain damage and certain neuropsychological disorders; it has been found to interfere with normal endocrine system development and function; and it depresses the immune system. It also presents various liabilities to one's safety. If your alcohol intake already falls in the category of moderate, try decreasing it and see if you notice any positive effects.

Traditional Chinese medicine teaches that ED may be cured with meditation, a positive attitude, qi gong exercise, practical techniques, and a correct diet. Practitioners recommend refraining from smoking, drinking, and taking drugs; as well as from consuming saturated fats, caffeine, and sugar. Instead, consume foods high in protein and complex carbohydrates.

Walnuts are a particularly fine source of protein, and eating walnuts for ten days before bedtime is a traditional remedy for ED. You can try roasting the nut meats in a dry frying pan or wok for three minutes, then grinding them into a coarse powder. Or you may also eat ten raw walnuts every day for one month. Seafood and shrimp also improve sexual energy.

In addition, Chinese vegetables have been found to be quite beneficial for increasing sexual activity. For example, the leaves of daikon greens are often used in macrobiotic regimens for strengthening the sex organs. They are chewy, but can be softened and cooked with a bit of diluted miso; they also go well sautéed with fried tofu. Pickles can also be made of this vegetable.

More familiar vegetables are also worth eating in greater quantities. Broccoli has been known for years as a powerful food source, especially as an antioxidant; it seems to be good for just about all conditions and diseases. Few besides former President George Bush and some small children malign the beautiful, dark green vegetable. It is an excellent source of vitamins A and C, is a good source of folic acid, is rich in fiber, is a source of calcium and iron, and may help prevent cancer. Broccoli (and brussels sprouts) also contains glucosinolates, secondary compounds that have anticancer effects. Eating five servings of fruits and vegetables a day can prevent more than 20 percent of all cancer cases. As Neal Barnard, M.D., author of *Foods That Fight Pain* and *Foods for Life*, has said, "Lining up for broccoli is more important than lining up for Viagra."

Another popular vegetable that is available year-round and extremely healthy is the potato. Researchers have found that potatoes are second to broccoli in terms of certain beneficial qualities. Lab results showed that, on a scale of one hundred, broccoli had an antioxidant value of approximately ninety-six and potatoes one of about sixty-nine. One potato also contains a high amount of vitamin C and 750 mg of potassium and is high in dietary fiber and iron.

In addition to evaluating your diet for weaknesses and supplementing food intake with vitamins, you can also add nutritional snacks to your regimen. Naturopathic physicians, who are known for their holistic approach to health and their concern with nutrition, often recommend the following shake as a breakfast or snack during periods of overwork and fatigue that coincide with a decrease in sexual capacities. You can make "Dragon's Milk" in your kitchen blender by combining these ingredients:

> 10 ounces reduced fat or skim milk, or 10 ounces apple juice
> 1 tablespoon crushed almonds
> 1 tablespoon powdered brewer's yeast
> 1 tablespoon sesame seeds
> 1 tablespoon honey
> 1 tablespoon raw wheat germ
> 1 teaspoon powdered ginseng
> 1 splash of natural vanilla extract
> 1 pinch of cinnamon (optional)
> 1 banana (optional)

Blend well and drink immediately. You can also substitute soy or rice milk for cow's milk. This vitamin-packed shake is a great replacement for the rushed cup of coffee and nutritionally bankrupt doughnut that often accompany the average morning commute.

In general, a diet that is heavy on fresh produce and whole grains and light on meat and dairy products, both sources of saturated fat, can help keep arteries free of the plaque that chokes blood flow to both the heart and to the penis. Breakthrough clinical trials by Dean Ornish, M.D., revealed that a combination of a low-fat vegetarian diet, appropriate exercise, stress management, and cessation of smoking allowed arteries to clean themselves out in 82 percent of participants. The study also suggests that many other factors that contribute to ED—diabetes, obesity, and hypertension—can be influenced by a menu change. With the right food and adequate exercise, many men can eventually overcome ED and have happier sex lives.

VITAMINS

Medical researchers are constantly discovering how vitamins affect our health and are used by our bodies. Four of the vitamin Bs may be especially useful for sexual dysfunction, and adding a multi-B vitamin to your diet may be worthwhile. Brewer's yeast is rich in B vitamins and can be sprinkled on popcorn, soups, and sauces or mixed in casseroles. Vitamin B_3 may increase blood flow to the penis. Taken about thirty minutes before having sex, it may enhance the intensity of the orgasm as well. Vitamin B_5 supports adrenal function and provides pituitary support, thereby improving sexual stamina. Vitamin B_6 is related to making neurotransmitters, such as epinephrine, thought to be involved in orgasm. It also may help male sex drive and lessen ED. And vitamin B_{12}, found in healthy sperm, may help ease ED and support adrenal function.

Certainly, vitamin C is often called on for a plethora of reasons, among them the prevention and treatment of the common cold and flu. But vitamin C, also known as ascorbic acid, has also been touted as useful in the treatment of ED. Vitamins C and E, zinc, and essential fatty acids are necessary for normal male sexual function. All these substances, normally found in the prostate gland, are critical for sperm and seminal fluid production. Vitamin C is found most readily in citrus fruits, berries, melons, tomatoes, potatoes, green peppers, and all leafy green vegetables. Overcooking, processing, or storage can destroy vitamin C, which is highly sensitive to air, heat, and water.

If you choose to take tablets, the recommended daily allowance for adults is 60 mg in the United States; recommendations in other Western countries range from 30 mg to 75 mg. During stressful situations such as trauma, infection, strenuous exercise, and elevated temperatures, the body's need for vitamin C increases. Smokers should take 100 mg per day. High doses of more than 1,000 mg of vitamin C a day may cause gastrointestinal disturbances. If you get diarrhea, reduce your dosage. High dosages should generally be avoided in people with a history of renal stones or those with diseases related to excessive iron accumulation. Vitamin C is water soluble and must be consumed daily.

Vitamin C performs several functions, but is most recognized for the prevention and treatment of scurvy. It also may be linked to the prevention of cardiovascular diseases. It also plays an important role in the synthesis of neurotransmitters and steroid hormones.

Also considered useful in treating ED is vitamin E, or tocopherol, also known as "the reproductive vitamin." An essential fat-soluble vitamin, it includes eight naturally occurring compounds. In the body, vitamin E is found in greatest concentration in the anterior pituitary gland, where it positively influences the production of male sex hormones. It also protects these hormones and other body substances from oxidation. Although there is no evidence that vitamin E directly enhances male potency, it indirectly slows down premature aging. In this way, the vitamin may well prevent the loss of flexibility in the walls of penile erectile tissue.

Food sources include vegetables and seed oils such as soybean, safflower, and corn; sunflower seeds; nuts; whole grains; and wheat germ. Leafy vegetables are also good sources. Absorption of vitamin E is dependent on the digestion and absorption of fat.

Some studies indicate that vitamin E supplementation significantly improves immune response in healthy older people. Also, high serum vitamin E levels have been correlated with reduced risk for coronary heart disease in both men and women. A Health Professionals Follow-up Study of 39,910 male physicians found that those who took at least 100 IUs of vitamin E daily for a minimum of two years had 37 percent less coronary disease. In another study conducted in four U.S. regions, people who had at some time regularly taken vitamin E supplements had lower rates of oral and throat cancer.

The current U.S. RDA for men is 10 mg and 8 mg for women. The requirement for this vitamin increases with higher intakes of polyunsaturated fatty acids. To determine the ideal amount, one should consider one's age, intake of other antioxidants, exposure to environmental pollutants, and level of physical activity. Fortunately, vitamin E is relatively safe. Few side effects, even from high intakes, have been reported. The recommended dose is 400 to 1600 units taken daily. However, high dosages may be contraindicated when a coagulation defect is present because of vitamin K deficiency or in those taking anticoagulant drugs. Also, people with extreme high blood pressure or heat damage from chronic rheumatic fever should not take large amounts of this vitamin. The natural form of vitamin E is always preferable to taking the synthetic form.

The body needs zinc, an essential mineral, to keep the reproductive system healthy. Zinc is linked in the male body to the output of testosterone, and low levels of zinc may contribute to ED. This mineral is also important for various enzyme reactions and the manufacture of protein. People living near the Caspian Sea in Iran are known to experience a higher rate of sexual and hormonal difficulties due to diets deficient in zinc.

Zinc occurs naturally in animal tissues and in plants grown in rich soil. Red meat contains much more zinc than vegetables; beef, pork, and lamb all contain significant amounts. Oysters are one of the richest sources of zinc, which perhaps accounts for their reputation as an aphrodisiac. The plant foods highest in zinc content are bran, nuts, legumes (including peanuts), and green leafy vegetables, although the zinc in plant proteins is not as readily available to the body as that in animal proteins. Diets based largely on processed foods may not include enough zinc. If you prefer, you can take a supplement to be sure you are getting enough zinc; the U.S. RDA for adults is 15 mg of zinc. Be sure not to take megadoses of zinc because too much can be harmful. Doses between seventy and one hundred times the RDA can cause cramps, vomiting, and diarrhea.

Phosphorus, a mineral, is found naturally in every cell of our body; the greatest amount of it can be found in bone and in muscle. It often functions with calcium in the forming of calcium phosphate in the bones and teeth at a ratio of two to one. Phosphorus is important in the utilization of carbohydrates, fats, and protein for growth and repair of cells and for the production of energy. It stimulates muscle contractions and is essential in treating disorders of the teeth and gums. Stress is definitely one condition for which phosphorus may be beneficial, thus the connection to ED.

Dietary deficiency of phosphorus rarely occurs. However, some disease conditions—malabsorption, diabetes, alcoholism, and extreme stress—may be associated with depleted levels of phosphorus. Phosphorus deficiency can cause lack of appetite or, conversely, obesity. Irregular breathing, mental and physical fatigue, and nervous disorders can occur. Severe deficiencies can cause seizure, coma, and even death. If the phosphorus content of the body is high, calcium should be taken to maintain a proper balance of the two.

Phosphorus should be taken as it naturally occurs in food. Food sources rich in protein are also high in phosphorus. Examples include milk, cheese, meat, poultry, fish, eggs, legumes, and whole grains. The recommended average daily intake is about 1,500 mg for men and 1,000 mg for women. Homeopathic preparations of phosphorus are useful for mental fatigue and nervous exhaustion, relief of muscle cramps and pain, and possibly improved nervous conditions.

GETTING FIT

In a recent study that followed nearly 22,000 men over an average eight-year period researchers found that fitness may well be the ultimate key to good health and longevity. Multiple studies reveal that at least half of the deterioration in body function that science has historically blamed on aging can be due to a sedentary lifestyle. The wasting of muscle tissue, loss of strength and endurance, and increased blood pressure that often accompany the aging process are not an inevitable consequence of the passing of time. And the best news is that it is never too late to start exercising.

Studies from Norway support these findings. Two recent comprehensive studies on 2,014 healthy men between the ages of forty and sixty undertaken by Dr. Gunnar Erikssen and colleagues at the Central Hospital of Akershus in Nordbyhagen, Norway, showed that even small increases in fitness level were associated with significant reductions in the risk of early death. The men, who had no evidence of heart disease, cancer, liver disease, or other serious disorder, were first followed over a period of twenty-two years. They performed various exercise tests and filled out questionnaires. A second study was conducted from 1980 to 1982, targeting 91 percent of the same men who were still living. Three hundred twenty-eight had developed chronic diseases or could not complete all the tests, but the remaining still healthy 1,428 men were followed up until 1994. The overall study showed that regular exercise lowered the risk of early death. Not only did the men who exercised live longer on average, they also lived healthier lives. The researchers found that even moderate fitness programs helped add years to their lives.

To maximize the health benefits of exercise, you need to design a program that includes the right amounts of the right kinds of exercise and also fits into your lifestyle. A comprehensive exercise program need not take up an inordinate amount of time. Just be sure you combine aerobic activity, resistance training, and stretching as part of your routine. Aerobic exercise challenges our body to improve its energy production system, increasing levels of HDL cholesterol (the "good" cholesterol that reduces the risk of artery disease), more efficiently regulating blood sugar, and decreasing risk of blood clots. An added benefit of aerobic exercise is that it burns calories that might otherwise end up as fat. Resistance training creates denser bones, stronger muscles, and healthier joints. Studies indicate that older people who have a regular strength training program postpone age-related loss of muscle strength by an impressive ten to twenty years. Both aerobic exercise and resistance training must be preceded and followed by gentle, deep stretching, which increases flexibility and decreases joint pain.

Not all exercises fit all people. Not everyone likes prepackaged exercise programs like Jane Fonda tapes or aerobic classes in the company of twenty-some-things with Arnold Schwarzenegger muscles. There are a variety of more solitary aerobic exercises that, when done three to five times per week for twenty to sixty minutes per session, can help you lose weight, strengthen your heart muscles, increase your body's ability to use oxygen effectively, and, best of all, re-lieve stress. Can't find time? Make time. If you do, you will absolutely feel better.

A few activities that fall into the aerobics cat-egory are cycling, hiking, swimming, running, brisk walking, and tennis. All forms of cycling—mountain biking, road biking, stationary biking, or group cy-cling classes—provide a good aerobic workout. Other activities you can do by yourself include rowing, run-ning or jogging, inline skating or figure skating, stair climbing (take advantage of office and hotel stairwells); swimming or aqua aerobics; and, my personal favor-ite, walking. The best pace is one that keeps you in your target heart rate range for between twenty and sixty minutes. Aerobic exercise is good for you even at low intensities, but the rule of thumb is: the lower the intensity, the longer the workout. A twenty-minute session is fine if you are working at a high intensity (for example, jogging). If you choose a less intense activity such as walking, you will need to increase the length of your workout to perhaps forty to sixty minutes.

To find your target heart rate, you should first check in with your physician. The proper heart rate for aerobic training depends on age and current fitness level as well as on your overall physical health. The target heart rate zone keeps your heart beating at 55 percent to 85 percent of its maximum reserve. The goal is to maintain a level of about 75 percent of your heart's maximum reserve for at least twenty minutes. This level is optimal for developing and maintaining cardiovascular fitness, but you will probably want to aim much lower at first if you have been leading a sedentary lifestyle and work up to a higher level gradually. You can also make an appointment with a personal trainer to help you design a program of aerobic activity that will keep you challenged but not discourage you.

Walking is the easiest way to get aerobic exercise. Anyone of any size or age can safely do this at any time of the year. If you live in a climate with cold winters, find an inside track or get a treadmill—even a large shopping mall will do. You will be surprised how many others are there walking laps. Walking is low-impact and does not require expensive equipment or clothing. Wear supportive shoes and comfortably loose clothing. For a truly aerobic workout, monitor your heart rate by dividing your target heart rate range (appropriate beats per minute as determined by your physician or trainer) by six seconds, which will give you a count of beats per ten seconds. Thus you can take your pulse at your wrist or neck for ten seconds during your workout to see if you are within your optimal range. For the maximum effect, swing your arms, walk up and down hills, and turn the walk into a thorough workout. Walk with a friend or your partner for company and extra motivation.

Classes offer another opportunity to keep up your momentum. Aerobic ones range from hip-hop to step aerobics to stretching and more. Many classes follow a similar format: a warm-up session; an aerobic segment including knee lifts, leg kicks, and various dance movements; a cool-down during which you reduce your heart rate and blood flow; and a final muscle toning or strength training session. Exercises might include abdominal crunches or leg lifts, for example. Stretching should always be done after every muscle-toning exercise. Most people, even if reluctant to join aerobics classes, enjoy them once they have enrolled. A good workout is more rewarding than just sitting in a chair and watching television, and it's an immense stress reliever.

While aerobic exercise is critical to cut heart disease risk, control weight, improve blood pressure and mood, and relieve stress, building body strength is also important. In one study, ninety-year-old men who lifted weights boosted their muscular strength 174 percent in just eight weeks. Such activity slows the aging process while building muscles and bone density and increasing metabolic rate. The American College of Sports Medicine recommends that all adults do some strength training at least two times a week.

Weight training is best done after an aerobic warm-up and gentle stretching. Beginners should start with eight to ten exercises with free weights or weight machines. You can plan your program with the assistance of a trainer or a book on weight lifting. Be sure to cover the body's major muscle groups: legs, back, chest, shoulders, arms, and abdominals, and work from large muscle groups to smaller muscle groups. For example, work the chest first and the shoulders and arms second. Select a weight you can lift for twelve to fifteen repetitions per set. Rest for a few minutes and then complete another set or two. Maintaining the correct form is more important than lifting heavy weights. The last few repetitions should be challenging, but you should be able to complete all the exercises with smooth, controlled motions. Jerky, out-of-control motions will result in injury. Resistance training should be completed two or three times a week with a day of rest in between each session for the muscles to recuperate.

For those times when you are just too busy to take even a short break from a stressful and demanding job, take comfort in knowing that any exercise is better than none at all. Daily activity of many kinds can contribute to fitness and good health. If you can't make it to the gym more than once this week, compensate by taking the stairs instead of the elevator or playing soccer with the neighborhood kids. You can also literally run—or at least walk—to do your errands: jog to the bank or dry cleaners. Ride your bike to work once. Deep breathing is another highly portable exercise routine. Another is shaking various parts of your body. Shake arms and hands; legs and feet; your head and your shoulders. These simple actions will help relieve the stress of a long day and carry you through until you can resume your regular exercise program. The following chapter contains additional suggestions for creating a personal fitness and relaxation practice that will help reduce stress, strengthen the body, and renew your energy.

9 INTEGRATING BODY AND MIND

YOGA, MEDITATION, AND RELAXATION EXERCISES

This chapter provides some basic information about other alternative healing methods that you may want to incorporate into your lifestyle changes. As you examine ways to improve your sexual life with healthier foods, exercise, and herbs or perhaps sex therapy, you may want to explore how taking up yoga or a regular visualization practice can enhance your recovery. Many alternatives exist and the following chapter offers only a brief sampling of those that you may find most useful. Each one of these methods can be studied in more depth with a teacher or with a book that focuses exclusively on that practice (see the bibliography for some suggestions).

HATHA YOGA

Yoga is a technique for achieving spiritual control and relaxation of the body. The origin of yoga, which derives from the Sanskrit word *yug* meaning "union with the divine," goes back more than five thousand years. The term defines a union between body, mind, and spirit by way of a certain state of consciousness; it also covers the methods that are used to reach this state. In yoga the embodied spirit becomes one with the universal spirit through the regular practice of certain physical and mental exercises. Yoga is now recognized as beneficial for general health problems as well as for its preventive and curative effects for allergies, headaches, high and low blood pressure, and insomnia. Yoga is also extremely useful in the treatment of erectile dysfunction.

When we speak of yoga, we usually mean physical yoga exercises or *asanas*, as they are called in Sanskrit. Hatha yoga, which is well known in America as an exercise and stress-management system, combines postures with breathing, relaxation, diet regulations, and meditation. To experience the spiritual aspects of yoga the asanas must first be practiced until they can be done comfortably. Only then can the asanas change from a set of physical exercises to a form of meditation—and thence to an awakening of spiritual power.

Hatha yoga teaches you how to use, store, and promote the free flow of the life force (*prana*). Hatha yoga is not an end in itself, but rather a preparation for a higher spiritual yoga. The body is enlivened by positive and negative currents, and when these currents are in balance, they induce perfect health. In the ancient language of Sanskrit, *ha* represents the cool energy of the moon and *tha* that of the hot energy of the sun. The word *hatha* then contains both elements. Certain yoga postures are specifically recommended for sexual disorders because they balance the flow of energies required for healthy sexuality.

These asanas, if correctly prescribed for your specific constitution by an experienced teacher, should be easy and pleasant to practice—indeed the very word *asana* means "a comfortable, stable position." Yogis have discovered that certain positions can endow human beings with qualities they are lacking. The following asanas are special positions of the body that should balance the endocrine, nervous, and circulatory systems. They are especially beneficial for erectile dysfunction because they stimulate the endocrine glands.

If you have never practiced yoga, you may want to sign up for a hatha yoga class. There you can work with a teacher to design a personal practice that will fit your individual needs. The following postures are best incorporated into a practice that includes a balanced sequence of postures—standing, lying down, and inverted. A yoga teacher is especially suited to advise you about the order in which to practice your postures and how many times to repeat a posture. This will allow you to gain the maximum benefits from the asanas.

GUIDELINES FOR ASANAS

- It is best to perform the exercises early in the morning or in the evening before supper. Do not practice asanas on a full stomach. Wait at least two or three hours after a meal.
- While practicing asanas, make sure that the room is well ventilated and smoke-free.

- Most exercises should be performed with the eyes closed.
- Hatha yoga exercises should be performed on a mat over a hard floor, not on a soft sofa or mattress.

PAN-PHYSICAL POSE OR CANDLE POSTURE (SARVANGA ASANA)

This posture, a shoulder stand, consists of four parts and is one of the most important asanas. It benefits the entire organism and should be practiced several times daily.

Lying on your back, with your arms extended next to the body, palms on the floor, slowly inhale and lift your extended legs—without bending the knees—until your legs are vertically above you. As soon as you reach this position, raise the trunk so that your hips rest on your hands. From here, push your trunk upward until it and your legs are in a straight line vertically above you and your chin is pressed firmly against your chest. Breathing abdominally, remain in this posture as long as it is comfortable.

Beginners should only remain in this posture briefly and gradually increase its duration as they grow used to the position. To conclude the exercise, slowly lower the trunk and then your feet to the floor. Never collapse like a sack! Remain prone for a few seconds, breathing smoothly and uniformly, to allow the blood circulation to return to its normal channels.

Hatha yoga maintains that man in his normal upright posture receives negative currents through his feet and positive ones through his head. In this asana, the effect is the opposite, hence the therapeutic value of this exercise. Those organs that in normal life are in the upper part of the body are resituated in the lower during the execution of the posture.

At the same time, the lungs and all the other organs in the region of the neck are bathed by a flow of blood. By pressing your chin against your chest, you prevent an excessive rush of blood to your head; by means of abdominal breathing, you press the veins together so as to avoid congestion. The veins of the neck are nevertheless filled with blood so that the endocrine glands—thyroid, pineal, and pituitary—receive fresh nourishment. This could explain why sarvanga asana is so often recommended to treat erectile dysfunction.

The organs of the abdomen that are normally supplied with an abundance of blood—because the blood in flowing downward expands the blood vessels—are held above the other organs in the practice of the sarvanga asana. These abdominal organs are thus relieved of any excess of blood, causing the blood vessels to contract again and to recover their resilience. People suffering from varicose veins or hemorrhoids also find that the exercise of this asana has a miraculous effect, even if practiced for only a few minutes a day.

PLOW POSTURE (HALA ASANA)

This asana is called the plow posture because in it one resembles an old-style farm plow. The posture consists of three stages. People with an excessively stiff backbone should be cautious when beginning this exercise, but after a few weeks of diligent practice, the stiffest spine will become limber.

First phase: Lie on your back with outstretched arms, palms down beside the thighs. Exhale slowly and lift both feet; carry on beyond your head until your toes touch the floor. Hold your arms flat on the floor, palms down.

Second phase: Place your toes on the floor, near your head, pushing your feet much farther backward. Breathe deeply and try to keep your knees as stiff as you can. You will find that your weight shifts toward the top of the spine.

Third phase: Your weight is supported by the vertebrae of the neck, so that your entire spine takes part in this exercise. Push your feet—with knees stiff— still farther behind you, draw in your arms, and clasp both hands behind the neck. Remain in this position a few seconds, or for as long as possible without exertion, and then slowly "unroll" until your feet return to your starting position.

This asana has a rejuvenating effect on the sexual glands as well as on the pancreas, liver, spleen, kidneys, and suprarenal glands. It also has a beneficial effect on all the vertebrae, and in its various phases every part of the spinal column is subjected to compression or tension. In this manner, the blood circulation is thoroughly freshened, and a fresh blood supply brought to the most important nerve centers along the spine.

The plow pose also has a strengthening effect on the organs of the thorax and the region of the neck. The entire glandular system is rejuvenated, as are the glands of the brain. Headaches frequently disappear with continued practice.

FISH POSTURE (MATSYA ASANA)

Sitting on the floor, place the right foot on the left thigh and draw the left foot over the right one, placing it on the right thigh. This is the lotus posture. The farther back you bring the foot toward the abdomen, the easier the exercise will be.

With the help of your elbows, lower the trunk backward until, with your chest arching upward, the top of your head is resting on the floor. Grasp your toes with your hands. Breathe lightly and avoid even the slightest tension. The consciousness is directed toward the thyroid gland in the center of the neck.

This asana is highly recommended for ED and also for colds because it stimulates the thyroid and all the organs of the neck.

PINCER (PASHCHIMOTANA ASANA)

Beginners may find this posture difficult, but again, with practice the spine will become more elastic.

Lying on your back, raise your arms, inhaling deeply, until your arms are flat on the floor behind you. Then, breathing out, sit up slowly, bending forward until your fingers touch your toes or until you can grasp your ankles. Your knees must remain straight. Bend your head forward until it touches your knees (beginners should get as close as they can without straining), and your elbows rest on the floor. Breathing in deeply, sit up and lie back slowly on the floor, your arms at rest next to your body. Exhale and relax. Focus your consciousness steadily on your solar plexus.

The sexual organs—rectum, prostate, and bladder, together with their nerves—are abundantly supplied with blood when this asana is practiced, so their condition should be improved. This is why this posture benefits those with erectile dysfunction. Hemorrhoids, diabetes, functional disturbances of the stomach, liver, and intestines (constipation, diarrhea) are also be helped by this exercise.

CHI KUNG

Chi kung is a Chinese form of exercise based on movements that do not exert the muscles or increase heart or breath rate. In fact, breathing slows down. Chi kung is done in three positions: standing, moving (with a dancelike motion), and sitting. These exercises are useful for adults and children of all ages. For the elderly, chi kung relaxes the stiffened joints and improves energy circulation throughout the entire body. The practice is at least five thousand years old and is thought to have originated in China's Middle Kingdom. Other civilizations, such as the Incas, Egyptians, and Islamic cultures, have similar exercise forms.

Chi kung is especially useful for emotional and mental stress because it balances the forces of yin and yang in the body, opening the way for renewed energy and strengthening your mental and physical powers. Two especially effective exercises for men, both of which strengthen vital jing energy, are called Embracing the Tree and Eight Pieces of Brocade. There are too many steps involved in these exercises to fully explain them here, but men who are interested can find them in Yves Réquéna's book *Chi Kung*.

The exercises take only half an hour a day and can radically improve your health and well-being. Beginners should wear loose-fitting, comfortable cotton clothing and remove jewelry and glasses before exercising. Bare feet will give you a good grip on the ground or floor but socks may be needed in chilly weather. Face south or east or toward an open window, and practice in a calm environment. Wait at least an hour after eating before practicing. Many communities offer classes or workshops on the techniques; no fancy equipment is necessary; and many of the exercises can be done outside.

ACUPUNCTURE

Acupuncture is a traditional system of medicine that was developed in China five thousand years ago. Traditional Chinese medicine (TCM) views the healthy human being as one who is living in harmony with the universe. Our being derives from the breath of the skies and the earth. All aspects of life are interrelated and body, mind, and spirit cannot be separated.

The basic theory of TCM is that the body consists of two opposing energies, yin and yang. Yin energy is passive, cool, dark, and feminine; yang energy is stimulating, hot, bright, and masculine. Human energy runs along main circuits called meridians, imaginary lines linking the organs (liver, lungs, heart, spleen, kidneys) and the intestines (stomach, small and large intestines, gallbladder, and bladder). According the theory of acupuncture, all diseases originate in a disruption of energy circulation and an imbalance of yin and yang. By using small needles to redirect and correct the body's flow of energy, acupuncturists can cure specific conditions and restore the body to its natural state of health.

Acupuncture is therapeutic for a wide variety of sexual dysfunctions. Loss of libido, erectile dysfunction, and premature ejaculation can often be treated successfully by a professional practitioner. The medical examination carried out by an acupuncturist differs considerably from that practiced by western physicians. Acupuncture employs no drugs and covers a scope much wider than that of western medicine.

An acupuncturist will begin by taking your full medical history and will examine your appearance and color. He or she may examine your eyes, skin, and tongue and will take as many as fourteen pulses. Once a diagnosis has been determined, the acupuncturist will insert several very fine needles into different body parts where they will be left for about half an hour. The needles are so fine that they hurt only briefly at the moment of insertion. (Do not worry that needles will be inserted into any sensitive areas—the acupuncture points on the body that heal the genitals are not on the penis!) Sometimes moxa (a stick of dried mugwort) may be burned to transmit heat to the skin. It will not touch your skin directly. Other times suction cups may be applied to the back.

After a treatment you may feel tired or a bit lightheaded. Be sure to take the time to rest and relax.

Acupuncture frequently proves to be effective when orthodox treatments have failed and is certainly worth trying. You can also try massaging acupuncture pressure points at home. The following two exercises are recommended to stimulate sexual energy.

Both should be performed several times in succession on a regular basis. You should be naked for both exercises.

1. In a standing position, hold the penis in the left hand, exposing the crease on the right side of the groin. With the right hand, massage the right groin crease with a back-and-forth motion thirty-six times. Repeat the massage on the left side with the left hand. Press fairly hard as you massage. If the friction of your hand on the skin is uncomfortable, apply a little almond oil or baby powder to the area before massaging it.

2. This massage should be performed standing in front of a mirror. With the palm of the right hand, press the point half-way between the navel and the penis, along the median line of the body. The correct point should be one hand-width directly below the navel. Hold the pressure for a few seconds. The penis should rise when pressure is put on this point.

RELAXATION METHODS

Medical science is just beginning to discover what alternative practitioners have long known: relaxation offers the potential for powerful physical healing. A number of relaxation techniques are in common use today, and those suffering from ED may find them helpful on multiple levels. For ED with physical causes, relaxation provides a much-needed break from the stress of living with ED and perhaps other serious health concerns. For ED with primarily psychological roots, relaxation methods can even reduce stress levels enough to resolve the problem entirely. The common goal is to achieve whole-body relaxation through codified exercises. Just as exercise programs are not one-size-fits-all propositions, relaxation practices are a personal choice. You may wish to try several different methods before settling on the one that works for you.

THE SCHULTZ METHOD

Relaxation can be achieved by learning to experience fully the sensations of heaviness and heat, according to the Schultz method. This approach starts off with a training session run by a professional therapist; the patient can later practice the method on his own. The patient is treated lying down with his eyes closed. The therapist instructs the patient to look for a feeling of heaviness on a particular area of his arm. The therapist then suggests the spread of muscular relaxation throughout the arm. Between sessions, the patient regularly practices exercises in which certain muscles are tensed and then relaxed. Additional techniques of respiratory, abdominal, and cardiac regulation enhance the therapist's verbal suggestions.

The next stage involves mental exercises, in which the patient learns to reproduce shapes, colors, and thoughts that have strong affective connotations. For instance, the patient lies down in a quiet place, closes his eyes and imagines himself stretched on a white sandy beach under a coconut tree somewhere in the Pacific. He visualizes ideas such as "I am completely calm" or "my arm is completely heavy." Eventually he will attain a state of total muscular relaxation and, once he has mastered the technique, a restful feeling of mental detachment. The Schultz method is especially useful for those who have never tried any visualization or relaxation techniques on their own and who find it difficult to concentrate long enough to relax fully.

BREATHING EXERCISES

Proper breathing is crucial to relaxation. Here are two breathing exercises to be carried out regularly, in an atmosphere of quiet.

Abdominal breathing

Lie on your back and place a heavy book or a telephone directory on your belly. Exhale slowly and thoroughly while sucking your stomach in as far as possible. When you feel the need to inhale, do so slowly and inflate your stomach not just the top of your chest. With your lungs full, hold your breath; exhale as soon as this becomes uncomfortable. You should always inhale and exhale through your nose. Try, very gradually, to slow down your rate of breathing and deepen your inhalation and exhalation.

Alternating nostril breathing

Alternate nostril breathing is a technique with its roots in yoga. Sit in a cross-legged position. If you can comfortably assume the lotus position (cross-legged with your feet resting on the opposite thigh), do so but do not stress your legs if you cannot. You can also sit on your knees or in a chair. Any comfortable position in which you keep your spine erect but relaxed is fine.

Close the left nostril with the left index finger. Draw in a deep breath through the right nostril. Hold this for a short while, then breathe out through the right nostril. Keep your lungs empty for a short while, then swallow your saliva. Release the left hand and close the right nostril with the right index. Repeat the exercise again, alternating nostrils. The pauses with your lungs empty or full should be of equal length. Gradually, you should be able to increase this length of time. Take six breaths, then rest for two minutes; then take six more breaths.

MEDITATION

While meditation can be part of a spiritual practice, it can also be used to promote relaxation and healing. Many people think of meditation as a rather elaborate set of mind-training exercises, but a meditation practice need not be complicated. A simple definition of meditation is intentional awareness. While meditation cannot wipe away all stress from our lives, it can help us deal more calmly and effectively with stressful situations. Perhaps best of all, it requires no special training or equipment, although group or private classes certainly can be beneficial.

There are as many ways to meditate as there are people who meditate, and you can also refer to numerous books that contain more detailed suggestions for creating a personal practice. A classic exercise is to sit or kneel comfortably in a quiet environment—any position in which you are alert and your spine is straight will do. Focus your attention on your breath. Looking at the flame of a candle or at a calming and beautiful image can help you center yourself and awaken mindfulness. Breathe naturally but focus your attention as you exhale. Imagine that all the difficulties you face in life are being dissipated with each outbreath. There will be a pause before you inhale again; just rest for a moment in that gap between breaths.

It may be difficult at first to simply "watch" your breath and not get caught up in the racing of your mind. But with additional practice, you will find that first a few seconds and eventually a few minutes will pass with your mind resting in its stillness. There is no right amount of time to meditate. A few mindful minutes are far better than struggling to sit for twenty or thirty minutes, and taking only five minutes a day to meditate is more beneficial than putting it off and trying to make up for lost time with one long weekly session.

VISUALIZATION

Visualization, which can also be practiced in any quiet moments during your day, harnesses the healing potential of mental imagery. Often we have trained our minds so well to produce negative and alarming images that we can no longer automatically conjure up positive ones. The stress and anxiety that result from experiencing ED provide a perfect example of how this can work: once you begin to see ED as inevitable, you may find your mind dwelling on what will go wrong during your next sexual encounter. When you prove yourself right, you reinforce the negative image. And yet the links between our minds and the physical health of our bodies are so strong that we can often reverse the process by changing the image.

Visualization differs from wishful thinking in its intent and focus. Visualization consists of consciously projecting images of the desired goal. The earliest records of this healing technique date back to ancient Babylonia and Sumeria. While visualization can be used for simple relaxation (for example, by taking time each day to imagine unwinding on a sunny beach), it can also be used to affect changes in involuntary body systems, increasing blood flow to the penis.

The most essential element of a visualization program is persistence. Visualization is a skill that takes practice. You might start by setting aside fifteen minutes a day to sit comfortably and quietly and imagine yourself having a successful sexual experience. Others may find it more helpful to look at an anatomy book, read a description of what happens physically to create an erection, and then imagine the different body parts functioning perfectly. Some people imagine energy as a color or blood as sensation of warmth flowing through a particular body part. You can also mentally repeat a sentence during your session such as, "Blood is rushing to my penis." Once you have practiced seeing the same positive image in your mind and can repeat it at will, you can take a few moments throughout the day to visualize it again.

If you have difficulty putting together a practice independently, you can seek the assistance of an autogenic trainer. This method is the most fully researched and widely used visualization method for healing. It has long been popular in Europe and is gaining popularity in the United States in stress-management programs. A practitioner will guide you through the process, and you will eventually be able to continue on your own.

EXERCISES FOR RECOVERY

As you continue on the path toward a renewed sexuality, spontaneous erections will begin to reappear and, with a little stimulation, the penis will again function normally. Here are two exercises that will help a man on the way to recovery get used to renewed tumescence. These exercises are centered on the voluntary control of the sphincter muscle. Once regular erections have been restored, these exercises can be practiced regularly to ensure better control over ejaculation.

The Kegel is a simple exercise commonly used to prevent urinary incontinence and by pregnant women preparing for birth. The basic technique is to repeatedly contract and relax the muscles in the pelvis that are used to interrupt urination. Practice holding for ten seconds and then releasing. A set consists of five to eight repetitions. You can easily and conveniently complete several sets during the day (for example, standing in line at the bank or waiting in traffic).

When performed regularly, Kegels can help you tone these all-important muscles. In a study released in 1993, men with ED due to leaking veins found Kegel exercises almost as effective as surgery in restoring erections. Forty-two percent of the patients who completed the training program were satisfied with the outcome and refused surgery.

This variation on the Kegel exercise requires an erection. With the penis erect, stand up and hang a towel on the penis. Try to lift it a dozen times in succession by contracting and relaxing the sphincter muscle.

HYPNOTISM

Hypnotherapy has been occasionally used as one possible therapy treatment in cases of erectile dysfunction. This therapy was introduced by Franz Mesmer, an eighteenth-century Austrian working in Vienna. Coining the term "animal magnetism" to describe his work, Mesmer moved to Paris in 1778 and began treating his patients by putting them into a bathlike structure lined with iron filings and magnets. People from all over Europe came to his clinic, but the French Academy decided to investigate him in 1784. Benjamin Franklin, chemist Antoine Lavoisier, and Dr. Guillotin, inventor of that efficient killing device, took part in the investigation, which may have been the first controlled clinical trial. Mesmer was ultimately denounced as a fraud, but his success, based on his bedside manner rather than on his magnets, formed the basis of modern hypnosis, and was also responsible for the word *mesmerize.*

Hypnosis became more valued as a therapeutic tool around World War I, when a German analyst, Ernst Simmel, used it along with psychodynamic techniques. It was endorsed by the American Medical Association in 1958, but it has never been entirely legitimized. Hypnosis has been used to treat many conditions including migraines, obesity, addictions, cancer, low self-esteem, and ED.

Only about 5 to 10 percent of the human population is highly receptive to hypnosis. A few are so amenable that they can undergo surgery with only hypnosis and no drug-related anesthesia. Twenty-five to 30 percent are minimally susceptible, and everyone else falls somewhere in the middle. Trust between the therapist and the patient is certainly critical. Some people have fears about going under and never returning to the same world.

In a 1991 Australian study a thirty-eight-year-old man with ED was treated hypnoanalytically. The therapy was used to uncover his inhibitions, to elicit and release hidden emotions, to positively reframe his previous negative sexual experiences, and to strengthen his ego.

MUSIC

For centuries, music has been an intrinsic, necessary part of daily life for many of the world's people. From Gregorian chant to Keith Jarrett's piano solos, music can soothe us, slow us down, perk us up, change our mood, or enhance our productivity. According to Hal A. Lingerman, author of the *Healing Energies of Music*, "While the greatest pieces of music will energize and inspire all levels of your being, there are musical works that may appeal more specifically to certain parts of your makeup." Lingerman suggests that some music activates us physically and makes us stronger, while other compositions or recordings influence feelings and emotions. Other music may inspire us with new ideas and renewed creativity.

In his book, Lingerman gives specific titles of musical pieces that can help in certain situations. Although he does not specifically mention erectile dysfunction, he does mention several conditions that might be related: tension, hyperactivity, depression, fear, and grief. Here are some of his recommendations for tension or hyperactivity: J.S. Bach, Air on a G String; Pachelbel, Canon in D; Vivaldi, Flute concertos from the *Four Seasons*. For depression, fear, and grief: Haydn flute quartets; Sousa marches; Debussy's *La Mer;* Handel's *Water Music;* For strength and courage: Elgar's *Pomp and Circumstance,* March no. 1; Brahms, Symphony no. 2 (final movement); the "Star-Spangled Banner," or other national anthems.

Certain pieces affect the heart center and increase the flow of love energies. Such music often emphasizes the high strings of the orchestra, the harp, and the organ. Examples here include: Mozart, "I Shall Love Her"(an aria); Vaughan Williams, "Serenade to Music"; Linda Ronstadt, "Canciones de mi Padre"; J. S. Bach, "Jesu, Joy of Man's Desiring." Personal experimentation will reveal which pieces work best for you.

10 STRANGERS IN THE NIGHT

RELATIONSHIP FACTORS AND SEX THERAPY

Whether or not an erectile dysfunction has physiological roots, the reality of the problem will have psychological ramifications. In some cases if the physical problem is solved, the psychological problem will disappear on its own; more often, there are lingering issues and problems to be dealt with. And for the majority of men with erectile dysfunction who are part of a couple, the problem has affected the sexual and emotional lives of *two* people. This is why, to restore a healthy sexual relationship to a couple, it can be so helpful for both members to consult a sex therapist.

THE ROLE OF THE SEX THERAPIST: TREATING THE COUPLE

Sexuality is often the most fragile and sensitive domain in the relationship of a couple and sexual problems may reveal a problem in the relationship or an unconscious conflict. Therapy, therefore, consists of translating the sexual problem into verbal language, which often improves the problem.

In most cases, the first time a man comes to consult a doctor about erectile problems, he comes alone. He is mortified with embarrassment. He feels responsible for the problem. Guilty. He thinks that his partner's presence at the sex therapy consultation is not necessary. Many men tend to fault themselves for their erectile dysfunction, even in cases undoubtedly caused by physical problems over which they have little control.

In fact, the interaction between partners is an extremely important element in the history and the treatment of a sexual dysfunction. Sex is an act between two people, thus there is no sexual problem that does not concern the partner. The overall objective of treating ED, then, should be the enhancement of sexual satisfaction for both parties. To achieve this, restoration of erectile function alone is not always sufficient. The problem may have begun with some unhealthy dynamic between the partners, or some other problem may have created new tension for the couple. Whatever the case, the sex therapist will certainly encourage the patient to bring his partner to the ensuing sessions, and she must be actively involved in the treatment. Many treatment failures can be traced directly to partner resistance. The therapist's role is not to repair a mechanical breakdown, but to restore the patient's and his partner's ability to love and to make love. The patient, in sex therapy, is the couple, not the man or the woman separately. The therapist will listen to the partner, who will play her part by offering information, as well as her perceptions of the diagnosis and the different therapeutic possibilities. The more involved she is, the more she will involve her partner and the better their therapeutic chances will be.

ED is only a symptom of other problems, and it is crucial to try and understand its psychological component. The sexual symptom is often present as a defense mechanism to neutralize a subconscious conflict that frequently has nothing to do with the patient's sex life. A psychological barrier is preventing the penis from working properly. This may indicate a communication problem between partners. It may be the result of a conjugal disagreement. At the consultation, the man and even his partner may declare that there isn't the slightest conflict or problem betweeen them, apart from ED. In this case the trained therapist's role is to help the couple verbalize the conflicts they are repressing.

Sex therapists can play a valuable role even in cases in which a patient has regained erectile function with the use of Viagra. In the short term, the patient's immediate recovery of erectile capacity enables him to break the vicious circle of performance anxiety. He no longer fears another failure in advance and is reassured about his own manhood. However, though it is never reported amid the flood of Viagra success stories in the media, the patient, while perfectly able to achieve an erection with the help of a pill, sometimes feels a certain lassitude and has difficulties actually making himself use the pill. He sees no point in having sex because he still sees himself as a failure in terms of his masculinity because he is totally dependent on a pharmaceutical treatment. He is unable to express his virility himself, and this troubles him.

This situation exemplifies the limits of pharmaceutical treatments for erectile dysfunction. The man still has no sexual confidence, and the pill is not the magic solution that the patient thought it was when the doctor first prescribed it for him. An "erection helper" is often a crutch. If the patient (with his partner) does not receive psychological assistance, serious sexual difficulties may persist. And at this point discontinuing the pharmaceutical treatment is not an option, because losing the ability to attain an erection again would be further proof that the man has no control over his own virility.

In cases of mixed physiological-psychological erectile dysfunction (and it can be argued that this is the vast majority of cases), cooperation between the patient's urologist and sex therapist is essential. The initial therapeutic effects of the erection enhancer are usually an excellent way to begin treatment, to give the patient hope and show him that a cure is possible, and guidance from a sex therapist from the beginning helps him to understand that reachieving erection is only phase one of his recovery treatment. As the patient's confidence returns, the vasoactive substance can be progressively phased out while continuing the sex therapy. The fear of failure will disappear little by little and the psychological causes will gradually be understood and analyzed, with an ensuing re-organization of the psychological defense mechanism.

Another side effect of artificial inducers of erection is that they can actually widen the sexual rift between a man and his partner. This is because the knowledge that the erection was "caused" by some foreign substance, rather than the man's pure desire for his partner, can make the sex act seem mechanical. The partner comes to view herself as merely the object for the man's sexual release. There is no mental excitement from fantasy, and emotional intimacy is wiped out. This is particularly true with intracavernous injections, or MUSE pellets, which do indeed produce an erection regardless of circumstance, but the perception of artificiality can be created by Viagra as well. In these cases, a sex therapist will work to help restore the patient's and his partner's capacity to cherish one another and to understand that each is doing their best to please the other. Once emotionally fulfilling sex has been achieved while using the treatment method, it is often possible to slowly phase out the substance. Fear of failure will diminish and eventually disappear.

Every couple is a unique case. After listening to the patient and his partner, the sex therapist will explain the part played by psychological events within the problem of erectile dysfunction. The sex therapist serves as a conduit through which the actual experiences of the two partners can be put into words.

Problems in interpersonal relationships often have a direct impact on the sexual functioning of a couple. Partners may feel rejected and resentful, particularly if the affected man does not confide his own anxieties. It can be difficult to perform sexually when negative feelings are harbored by both partners. Guilt is also commonly experienced; both partners blame themselves (and sometimes the other) for what they each perceive as personal failure. Tension and anger frequently arise within relationships that lack communication about sex.

By listening to the patient and his partner, the sex therapist hopes to enable each of them to express their experience, their suffering. Lack of communication is usually the key to most problems between couples, and this is especially true with sexual problems, because the topic is extremely personal and the associated embarassment tends to discourage people—especially men—from expressing their problems verbally. This is why the primary goal of the sex therapist is to get couples talking. By restoring communication, and in so doing revealing the ways in which the couple relates, the sex therapist will help them dismantle sexual anxiety, restore tenderness, relaxation, and pleasure, and discover any behavioral ruts they tend to fall into. It often happens, during a consultation of this kind, that each person discovers for the first time how the other really feels and how far he or she is prepared to get involved in genuine therapy in order to recapture the spark the relationship once had. Simply discovering how much one's partner cares can be the best therapy of all.

In addition to exploring and improving the psychosexual dynamics between the couple, the sex therapist can be an expert source of information for all their questions about sexuality, a subject still largely shrouded in myths, despite the liberated media. It is amazing how many people still have major misconceptions about sex, in regard to what is normal, desirable, and acceptable. Learning the truth about sexuality, and realizing that they are not aberrant or insufficent in any way, can go a long way toward eliminating a couple's sexual hang-ups.

Sex therapy employs many of the same basic principles as regular psychotherapy. The difference is that its approach is developed specifically for the treatment of sexual problems. The new sex therapies evolved from the work of Dr. William H. Masters, Dr. Virginia E. Johnson, and Dr. Helen Singer Kaplan. One aspect of the treatment is sensate focus exercises designed to progressively and slowly improve erection performance by showing couples how to enjoy sexual activity other than intercourse. Couples learn to caress each other and to communicate physically. This shifts the emphasis from performance to the mutual exchange of pleasure. Practicing at home, the couple then visits their sex therapist to report on their "homework." This process helps to transform sex from an anxiety-filled activity into an eagerly anticipated, highly pleasurable event.

Many new ideas have been incorporated and sex therapies are now based largely on psychoeducation and cognitive, behavioral, or analytical therapies. Sex therapy programs generally span fifteen to thirty sessions, involving both partners, and consist of homework assignments, therapy sessions, and possibly the use of books and videos.

BREAKING THE ROUTINE: SEDUCTION, COMPLICITY, AND SEX GAMES

The therapist, as mentioned, may provide information that can help to correct myths and to reverse misunderstandings that adversely affect sexual functioning. But information may not be enough. Some couples may simply be bored with their physical relationship, which has become routine. There is no longer any eroticism and seduction associated with the sex act. Fortunately there are ways of improving relationships without having to look elsewhere, and the therapist will try to reinject dynamism into the couple's sexuality. As many people have stated, the brain is by far the most important sexual organ in the body. All sex is, to a greater or lesser degree, dependent on fantasy and perception, so tapping into new springs of erotic fantasy can be just what couples need to shake them out of the doldrums. The recommendations that follow may seem obvious to some readers, but the purpose of this chapter is to explain precisely what a sex therapist is liable to tell patients who consult him or her about conjugal problems.

Everyone has noticed how sexual relationships can suddenly improve with a "formal" date. What happens? On such occasions, men and women prepare themselves with extra care. They bathe and perfume themselves, put on their best clothes, and in general make a special effort to be as attractive to the other as possible. They go out to a restaurant or the theater—something they don't do very often. Their evening is organized around the idea of something private and pleasurable, from which everyone else—including chil-

dren—is for once excluded. The couple can enjoy being seductive for themselves, for each other, and for
other people who may see them, and sex will provide
the climax of this sharing. Sex is in the air, tantaliz-
ingly postponed by deep complicity. In this atmosphere, sex will not feel routine, and the final sensual
experience is liable to be unusually satisfying.

Sometimes the sexual possibilities may need to
be broadened. The therapist might advise adding a
little innocent spice to a relationship that has become
too monotonous or ritualized. For example, the woman
might spend the day wearing no underclothes, with
the full knowledge of her partner. The unknowing
glances of other people will strengthen the erotic current between the two. To make love in some unaccus-
tomed place, with the delicious fear of discovery, may
also work. Locations should be changed frequently—
the kitchen, the bathroom, or the woods, a deserted
beach, a car, an empty compartment on a train.

Then there are all manner of kinky scenarios for
foreplay. The man could have his wrists or ankles
bound. Some may prefer erotic accessories, special
lingerie, fancy clothes. Pornographic videocassettes
or gadgets sold in sex shops can also be fun. Played
once in a while, such fantasy games and objects
present no perils, provided they do not erode mutual
respect. And if you think this sort of thing sounds
silly, that doesn't preclude trying it—laughter can be
an excellent aphrodisiac.

Caressing is, most obviously, an indispensable
preliminary to sex, postponing penetration while in-
tensifying the experience of pleasure by anticipation.
Every couple should learn to exchange lengthy caresses

before the final stage of lovemaking: blowing delicately on the skin, nibbling, licking, fondling, featherlight massage. Most of all, the imagination must be given free rein. Here are some additional tips:

- Harsh lighting or total darkness are to be avoided. A warm and intimate ambiance can easily be created by filtered lighting or candles. The sight of one's partner is central, after all, to erotic excitement; visual stimuli can be enhanced by the judicious placement of mirrors on the bedroom wall or ceiling.
- Then there is the extra delight of music, which can not only relax the lovers, but also influence the rhythm of their lovemaking.
- The positions of lovemaking should be varied, as required, to avoid any impression of monotony—which in the long term acts as a brake on freedom of impulse.
- Finally, there are certain purely practical tricks that can spectacularly improve the quality of lovemaking. For example, a pillow slipped beneath the woman's coccyx will help the man to thrust his penis deeper—and if he can find a way to brace his feet against a wall or bedpost, he will add more power and control to his motions and lessen the strain on his back muscles.

POSITIONS FOR INTERCOURSE

Depending on the man's and woman's morphology, some sexual positions may be more conducive to pleasure than others:

FOR A LONG PENIS

Both people adopt a standing position. One leans against a wall. The depth of penetration is lessened because the woman has to keep her legs together to hold the penis.

FOR A SMALL PENIS

The woman lies on her back and the man enters her in the missionary position. The woman draws her pelvis closer to the man's by crossing her legs around her partner's back. This reduces the length of the vagina and facilitates deep penetration.

FOR A THICK PENIS

A man with a thick penis can sometimes experience difficulty penetrating the woman's vagina, which may be difficult and painful for the woman. To alleviate this, the woman should squat on all fours and the man can penetrate her from behind. In this position, the vagina and the penis have the same orientation and penetration is made easier. Lubricating gels can also help.

FOR A NARROW VAGINA

The woman lies on her back. Her bent legs rest against the man's shoulders. By raising the pelvis, this position enlarges the opening of the vagina, while reducing its length. If the man's penis is a large one, he should enter the woman very slowly and gently to avoid hurting her.

DURING PREGNANCY

The man lies on his back with the woman astride of him. This allows her total freedom of motion. She rests securely on her knees and can decide on the depth of penetration and the rhythm of movement, be it to and fro, rotating, or swaying.

FOR PREVENTING PREMATURE EJACULATION

The following four positions are recommended:

- The man stands, supporting the woman, who hangs around his neck. The problem with this position is that it can only last for a short time unless the man is unusually athletic and muscular.
- The man lies on his back with the woman straddling his body, facing him, with her feet at his shoulders. The woman can then follow her own rhythm, which is generally slower than the man's. Her movements are thus confined to pelvic rotations. This position maintains the level of arousal but doesn't always lead to ejaculation.
- The woman lies on her side, and the man enters her from behind. This position is not tiring; it is not deep either, and like the previous one, will maintain a high pitch of arousal. To achieve a deeper penetration, the woman can lift her thigh and curve herself forward.
- The man sits on a chair or a stool, and the woman straddles him face to face. Penetration and motions are both limited.

FOR DELAYING EJACULATION

The classic missionary position is advisable for delaying ejaculation. Here, the small aperture of the vagina grips the penis tightly. This sensation is increased if the woman presses her thighs closer together.

HE SAID, SHE SAID

> "Yielding to a man, the woman puts a violin
> in the hands of a gorilla."
>
> Honoré de Balzac

The fact is that men and women have very different sexual needs, drives, and expectations. A woman may express her feelings toward her partner in a relatively continuous manner, rather than exclusively during sexual activity. For a woman there is great continuity between daily life and sexual intercourse. If there has been a fight in the middle of the day, the woman, in bed at night, may remember this conflict with great intensity. There will be no excitement if her partner wants to make love to her at that precise moment. In contrast to this, a man may only express his tenderness and love when he is engaged in sexual intercourse. He is able to forget his anger and his moods of the day. Thus there is already a fundamental misunderstanding between him and his companion before they have even started making love. He wants to be close to her—but she hasn't yet digested their latest dispute.

Hence the need for a therapist, to act as a neutral third party. The therapist makes no judgment in favor of the man or the woman. His or her function is to help the couple take stock of their difficulties and conflicts, with a view to restoring full communication.

The therapist can also help the male patient understand how female sexuality differs from his own, and vice versa. The erogenous process of a man tends to work more rapidly than that of a woman. It takes her longer to reach orgasm than it does him. If a man ignores this fact, he is likely to experience solitary pleasure—and leave his partner unfulfilled. The woman may imagine that she is unable to achieve orgasm, when in reality she merely has an incompetent partner. Most sexual disagreements arise from this problem, which men all too often know little about.

So the emergence of sexual failure in a man is sometimes traceable to his ignorance of female sexuality. While his potency was intact, he should have learned more about a woman's body in order to coordinate and control his movements, his caresses, and his ejaculation so that his partner could herself experience deep clitoral and vaginal pleasure, and the resentment that leads to sexual failure would never have arisen in the first place. In these cases, restoring communication can have a very positive effect.

Aging also takes its toll on sexual function. Postmenopausal changes in hormones cause many women to lose interest in sex or to experience reduced lubrication and sensitivity, making sex less pleasurable at best and painful at worst, and therefore making it an activity they avoid when possible. In a recent poll, fully 43 percent of women were found to have some sort of sexual dysfunction, ranging from true physical problems to little interest or little enjoyment. It may have been a blessing in disguise for many of these women, who no longer had interest in sexual activity, when their men lost the capacity as well. The fact that they no longer needed to "satisfy their husbands" may have been just fine with them, so revived erectile capabilities in their mates may be something they are not ready for. A sex therapist can help these couples work through their different levels of desire without becoming too emotionally charged, and can also suggest ways for these women to rediscover some of the pleasure in sex.

THE ROLE OF THE PARTNER

The partner plays a vital part in correcting sexual failure. So, it is very important that the partner be actively involved in the treatment of erectile dysfunction. Only in rare cases—through ignorance, inhibition, or a cruel temperament—do women actually inhibit the recovery of men with erectile dysfunction. Each case is unique, but I have seen variations on the following stereotypes more than once in my practice:

• The woman who is broadly ignorant about male sexuality. For her, an erection is something natural and she cannot imagine that a psychological block can prevent the penis from functioning properly. If her partner has a sexual failure, she believes that he no longer finds her desirable. She has little or no perception of the force of anxiety generated in a man by the experience of erectile dysfunction. In this case, the therapist's role is to give the woman the information about male sexuality that she lacks. He will explain that episodes of erectile dysfunction are relatively common in men's lives, and will help her to understand that a more supportive attitude would be reassuring for her partner.

• The woman who has a competitive, aggressive relationship with her partner and may actively mock his erectile dysfunction. A variation on this is women who do not hesitate to talk about conflicts during sexual intercourse, or else make invidious comparisons to ex-lovers, whom they tend to overestimate. Consciously or unconsciously, they twist the knife in the wound, and turn one failure into an obsession prior to each new bout of sexual intercourse. The symptoms of erectile dysfunction will generally quickly worsen in these cases, and the therapist should recommend that the couple reevaluate their relationship, at the very least.

• The woman who feels inhibited about making love. In spite of sexual liberation, there are still many women who feel this way. Often these women have had a very religious upbringing, where any hint of sexuality was prohibited. Even if these women have managed to overcome their background enough to engage in intercourse, they may insist on using only the conventional missionary position, believing any other position to be "sinful" or "deviant." The heritage of Judeo-Christian culture still plays no small part in our lives, and that culture has traditionally frowned on different, more "lascivious" positions for lovemaking. When denied the possibility of introducing variety into their lovelife, the man may become bored with the routine or feel that it has lost its eroticism, and an erectile dysfunction may result.

• The woman in whom the fear of pregnancy is a dominant concern during sex. Such contraceptive methods as coitus interruptus deprive male sexuality of part of its fulfillment and have been traced to psy-

chological erectile dysfunction. It is infinitely preferable, and safer in every way, to use contraceptives.

Fortunately, of all the aphrodisiacs imagined by man,
the best by far is woman herself. Most women are capable of very deep and loving understanding. Faced
with sexual failure, they minimize its importance. The
understanding woman knows that an episode of erectile dysfunction is normal with any man. She will make
light of the matter and hold tiredness, stress, and worry
entirely to blame. On no account does she call her
mate's virility into doubt. On the contrary, she does
her best to provide her own form of therapeutic care.
She takes this opportunity to prove that what matters
most to her—and hence to him—is their relationship.
With wise care and treatment, his episode of erectile
dysfunction will probably be quickly forgotten.

GUIDELINES FOR SELECTING
A SEX THERAPIST

Very few states license sex therapists, so the patient
must exercise caution and must choose wisely. Individuals offering services related to sexual problems include psychiatrists, psychologists, social
workers, religious counselors, hypnotists, and many
others. Psychiatrists, of course, are licensed physicians with medical degrees. In all states, licensing
laws control who can call themselves a psychologist
or a physician.

   If you need a sex therapist, you might begin by
consulting your family physician, gynecologist, or
urologist. Ask for a referral to someone your doctor

has used confidently in the past. The American Association of Sex Educators, Counselors, and Therapists (AASECT) is the largest national group that certifies sex educators, sex counselors, and sex therapists. AASECT maintains a national register and can provide assistance in finding a qualified sex therapist in your area. Contact information for AASECT is listed in the resource section of this book.

Appendix

Frequently Asked
Questions about
Sexual Dysfunction

Is it desirable that one's partner should be present at a consultation for an erectile dysfunction?

Not necessarily. A woman does not usually bring her husband when she goes to see a gynecologist, and a man must be able to consult a doctor alone. However, if it is determined that relationship issues are involved in the ED, then it is essential that the partners visit the sex therapist together.

Is there a difference between ED and sterility?

ED and sterility have nothing in common. Patients with erectile dysfunction are usually still fertile. Sterility is due to an anomaly in the quantity or quality of the spermatozoa contained in the semen at the time of ejaculation. A sterile man has normal erections; his ability to have sex is not altered, while a man with ED finds it impossible to have normal sexual intercourse under normal circumstances.

Can one cure an erectile dysfunction that has existed for a long time?

Although a cure cannot be guaranteed, more often than not we can improve the quality of a man's erections, even if many years have passed since the onset of ED.

If a man experiences a tempory loss of erectile capability, is this considered an erectile dysfunction?

Absence of an erection can happen to any man one day or another. This can be explained by fatigue, a lowering of desire, an evening of too many drinks, or the stress of a new relationship, and is nothing to worry about. However, if the condition persists and interferes with a man's normal sexual activity, medical advice should be sought.

Are men over the age of seventy too old to benefit from today's treatments for ED?

No, it is never too late. A man is never too old to enjoy sexual pleasure.

What can a man do to reduce the risk of erectile dysfunction?

Living a healthy life can be good for the sex life. Avoid cigarettes, high-fat foods, and excessive alcohol consumption. In some cases, ED can be related to diabetes or other diseases. Visiting a doctor regularly will help to identify these problems as soon as possible.

Does having only one testicle lead to ED?

The testicles are formed in the belly of the male fetus before birth. They move progressively down the sides of the groin, eventually settling in the scrotum. Sometimes only one testicle makes its appearance before puberty; in this case medical treatment or surgery may be needed to bring down the other. If this fails, which it sometimes does, the adult man will have a half-empty scrotum, but his sex life will be perfectly normal. As a rule the production of spermatozoa from a single testicle is more than sufficient for impregnation.

Does a prostate operation invariably result in ED?

A prostate operation will result in sterility and in what is called a retrograde ejaculation, but the man will not have ED. Sex and orgasms are still possible, but the ejaculation is no longer projected outward; instead it is driven back into the bladder. The sperm is thenceforth evacuated with the urine.

In certain cases, the complete removal of the prostate may induce nervous lesions that provoke erectile dysfunction. In these conditions, an intracavernous injection treatment is the best method to restore erections.

I have difficulty ejaculating while having intercourse. Why is this?

During sexual intercourse, some men are unable to ejaculate, or they have a delayed ejaculation. This symptom can be psychological, but it is also a common side effect of medical treatments for anxiety and depression.

What is a man's ejaculate made of?

The chemical composition of ejaculate varies from individual to individual and within the same individual from time to time. Semen is essentially seminal plasma and spermatozoa. It contains minute quantities of more than thirty compounds such as fructose, ascorbic acid, cholesterol, creatinine, citric acid, sorbitol, pyruvic acid, glutathione, inositol, lactic acid, nitrogen, vitamin B_{12}, and various salts and enzymes. The average ejaculate also contains between 80 million and 800 million spermatozoa. The amount of ejaculate varies among men and the volume of any given man's ejaculate relates to his number of recent orgasms—the more orgasms, the lesser the amount of ejaculate; the average is one teaspoon of semen per orgasm. The caloric content of a teaspoon of semen is minimal, perhaps one or two calories, and the nutritional value is practically nonexistent.

What is a normal frequency of ejaculation?

According to a number of studies, many adolescent young men ejaculate daily, if not more frequently than that. This frequency gradually declines for most males to 2–3 times per week, which is typical of men in their forties. But there is considerable variation among men of all ages.

Can an ejaculation be painful? Is the presence of blood in the semen a cause for serious concern?

Normally ejaculation is not painful, though a few patients do complain about testicular pains. Pain when ejaculating is often due to a urogenital infection, causing traces of blood to appear in the sperm. This symptom may also occur in periods of overtiredness. The bleeding originates in the seminal vesicles, and its cause is unknown. The symptom may last two to three weeks and may sometimes recur, in which case a special evaluation is recommended, to locate what may be a serious prostate problem or infection. But be reassured—this symptom is usually nothing to worry about.

How can premature ejaculation be treated?

One man out of three is liable to encounter this difficulty at one stage or another of his lifetime. Ejaculation occurs either after only a few thrusts or else before the penis is inserted into the vagina. The origin of this symptom is psychological. It can be treated with psychotherapy or with medical treatments such as alpha blockers and antidepressants. Yohimbe has also shown great promise in delaying ejaculation. Sex therapy techniques can also help to recondition sexual responses.

Can a hernia generate erectile dysfunction?

Scrotal and penile hernias require surgery but this will in no way alter the erectile capabilities of the penis.

What is phimosis?

Phimosis is an abnormal stricture of the corona that prevents the foreskin from drawing clear of the glans in the normal way. It can generate an infection. The treatment requires partial or total circumcision.

Does vasectomy affect erectile function?

No. Vasectomy is a simple surgical procedure that some men willingly ask for when they no longer want children. The surgery consists in the ligation of a section of the vas deferens situated in the scrotum. After the operation, sperm can no longer be expelled via ejaculation—but this prevents neither the ejaculation of seminal liquid nor the orgasm. It is theoretically possible to reverse a vasectomy within a few years of having the operation, but not thereafter. Men often store sperm samples at a sperm bank before the vasectomy, in case they change their mind and want to have additional children later.

Does circumcision alter sexual intercourse?

Circumcision in no way alters sexual behavior. A lot of false information exists on this subject.

Is the presence of blood vessels under the skin of the penis a normal occurrence?

Blood flow is what generates the erection of the penis. The presence of blood vessels under the skin is perfectly normal. Some men may notice veins on the skin of their penis; this is also normal.

Should sexual activity be avoided when men have ED?

It is very important for men to continue to make love to their partner even if they cannot achieve a full erection. Stopping all sexual activity often means that a man and his partner feel less emotionally intimate and drift apart. Many women find kissing, caressing, fondling, and mutual masturbation at least as satisfying as sexual intercourse, if not more.

Is a penis that bends when erect abnormal?

The penis may bend when erect—this is quite normal. If the penis bends and there is pain during sexual intercourse, you may be suffering from Peyronie's disease. See the section in this book on Peyronie's disease for more information.

Can a woman have sexual intercourse during pregnancy?

Sexual intercourse with a pregnant woman is not only possible but also highly agreeable. Penetration does not traumatize the fetus in any way.

Does tobacco affect erectile capability?

Yes. Nicotine has a negative effect on erections by provoking the contraction of the vessels that bring the blood into the corpora cavernosa of the penis. High tobacco consumption is also a definite risk factor for atherosclerosis (hardening of the arteries). Men's sexual arteries are ideal targets for this disease, which results in erectile dysfunction.

Does obesity affect erectile capabilty?

Not directly, but it is associated with atherosclerosis and diabetes, both of which cause ED.

BIBLIOGRAPHY

GENERAL BIBLIOGRAPHY

Aaron, C. *Garlic Is Life.* Berkeley, CA: Ten Speed Press, 1996.

Acuff, R.V. "Get the Facts on Natural Vitamin." *Nature's Impact*, Feb./Mar. 1999, p. 29.

The American Journal of Hypertension. Vol. 11, Nov. 1998, pp. 1244–1247.

American Journal of Natural Medicine. Vol. 1, no. 3, Nov. 1994, p. 8.

American Psychiatric Association. *Diagnostic and Statistical Manual of Mental Disorders* (4th ed.). Washington DC: APA, 1995.

The Australian Journal of Clinical Hypnotherapy and Hypnosis. March 1991.

Barnard, N., and S. Chaitowitz. "To Heck with Viagra . . . I'll Have Spaghetti." Commentary for Physicians Committee for Responsible Medicine. Washington D.C., June 1998.

Beauvoir, S. de. *The Second Sex.* New York: Knopf, 1952.

Camphausen, R. C. *The Encyclopedia of Erotic Wisdom.* Rochester, VT: Inner Traditions International, 1991.

Culpepper, N. *The English Physitian.* London: Peter Cole, 1652.

Daniélou, A. *The Phallus*. Rochester, VT: Inner Traditions International, 1995.

De Luca, D. *Botanica Erotica*. Rochester, VT: Healing Arts Press, 1998.

Dening, S. *The Mythology of Sex*. New York: Simon and Schuster, 1996.

"Doctors Seek More Research on Erection Supplement." *New York Times Syndicate*, Feb. 15, 1999.

Dreyfus, E. A. "Sexuality and Sex Therapy." *Self-help and Psychology*, an on-line magazine at shpm.com, 1999.

801 Prescription Drugs: Good Effects, Side Effects and Natural Healing Alternatives. Peachtree City, GA: FC&A Publishing, 1996.

Ellis, A., and A. Abarbanel. *The Encyclopedia of Sexual Behavior*. New York: Jason Aronson, 1973.

"Exercise, Not Diet, Is Key to Healthy Living, Study Says." *New York Times Syndicate*, Mar. 5, 1999.

Foster, S., and Y. Chongxi. *Herbal Emissaries: Bringing Chinese Herbs to the West*. Rochester, VT: Healing Arts Press, 1992.

Frazer, Sir J. G. *The Golden Bough*. New York: Macmillan, 1963.

Fugh-Berman, A. *Alternative Medicine:What Works*. Tucson, AZ: Odonian Press, 1997.

Fulder, S. *The Book of Ginseng*. Rochester, VT: Healing Arts Press, 1993.

Gebhard, P. H., and A. B. Johnson. "The Kinsey Data: Marginal Tabulations of the 1938–1963 Interviews Conducted by the Institute for Sex Research." Philadelphia: W.B. Saunders, 1979.

"Go Heavy on the Veggies to Prevent Cancer." *New York Times Syndicate*, June 28, 1999. www.intelihealth.com.

Goldfinger, S.E. "Prevention." *Harvard Health Letter,* Vol. 24, 16, Mar. 1999.

Goldstein, I., and L. Rothstein. *The Potent Male.* Los Angeles: The Body Press, 1990.

Grady, D. "Sure, We've Got a Pill for That." *New York Times,* Feb. 14, 1999, section 4, page 1.

Grape, C.E. *Reproductive Biology of the Great Apes.* New York: Academic Press, 1981.

Griffin, G. *Penis Size and Enlargement.* Aptos, CA: Hourglass Book Publishing, 1995.

Hammond, W. *Sexual Impotence in the Male.* New York: Bermingham, 1883.

Harris, L.J. *The Book of Garlic, Revised Edition.* Los Angeles: Panjandrum/Aris Books, 1979.

Haynes, K. "The Viagra Alternatives." *Vegetarian Times,* issue 254, Oct. 1998, p. 26.

"The Healthy Diet." Johns Hopkins Health Information, www.intelihealth, June 26, 1999.

Henderson, C.W. "Viagra Makers Block Sex Drink 'Viagrene' in Britain." *Impotence and Male Health Weekly Plus*, Feb. 15, 1999.

Hite, S. *Hite Report on Male Sexuality.* New York: Alfred A. Knopf, 1981.

Hoffmann, D. *The Complete Illustrated Holistic Herbal.* Rockport, MA: Element Books, 1996.

Kaplan, H.S. *The New Sex Therapy.* New York: Brunner/ Mazel, 1974.

———. *The Illustrated Manual of Sex Therapy.* New York: Brunner/Mazel, 1975.

———. *How to Overcome Premature Ejaculation.* New York: Brunner/Mazel, 1989.

Keuls, E.C. *The Reign of the Phallus*. New York: Harper and Row, 1985.

Kinsey, A. C., W. B. Pomeroy, and C. E. Martin *Sexual Behaviour in the Human Male*. Philadelphia: W.B. Saunders, 1948.

Koldony, R.C., W. H. Masters, and V. E. Johnson. *Textbook of Sexual Medicine*. Boston: Little Brown, 1979.

Krane, R. J., M. B. Siroky, and I. Goldstein. *Male Sexual Dysfunction*. Boston: Little Brown, 1983.

Kumar, S. "Indian 'Me-Too' Drugs Could Pose Threat to Viagra." *Lancet*, vol. 351, issue 9117, 1998, p. 1712.

LeGrandPre, R. *Ritalin Nation: Rapid-Fire Culture and the Transformation of Human Consciousness*. New York: Norton, 1999.

Lehman, P. *Running Scared: Masculinity and the Representation of the Male Body*. Philadelphia: Temple University Press, 1993.

Levinson, D. J. *The Seasons of a Man's Life*. New York: Alfred A. Knopf, 1978.

Lingerman, H. A. *The Healing Energies of Music*. Wheaton, IL: Quest Books, 1995.

Lopiccolo, J., and L. Lopiccolo. *Handbook of Sex Therapy*. New York: Plenum Press, 1978.

MacKenzie, E., and B. MacKenzie. *It's Not All in Your Head*. New York: E.P. Dutton, 1989.

Malinowski, B. *Sex, Culture and Myth*. London: Hart Davis, 1963.

Marion, M. "An Alternative to Viagra." *Men's Health*, vol. 14, issue 1, Jan/Feb. 1999, p. 24.

Masters, W. H., and V. E. Johnson. *Human Sexual Response*. Boston: Little Brown, 1965.

———. *Human Sexual Inadequacy.* Boston: Little Brown, 1970.

Masters, W. H., V. E. Johnson, and R. C. Koldony. *Heterosexuality.* New York: Harper Perennial, 1994.

Milius, S. "DNA Tests Find Phony Seal Penises." *Science News*, vol. 153, no. 1, Jan. 3, 1998, p. 6.

Miller, R. A. *The Magical and Ritual Use of Aphrodisiacs.* Rochester, VT: Destiny Books, 1993.

Morgenstern, S., and A. Abrahams. *Love Again, Live Again.* Englewood Cliffs, N.J.: Prentice Hall, 1989.

Parsons, A. *Facts and Phalluses.* New York: Saint Martin's Press, 1990.

Phillips, K. D. Texas A & M University Agriculture News Home Page: http://agprogram.tamu.edu, June 9, 1995.

Reid, D. P. *Chinese Herbal Medicine.* Boston: Shambhala, 1987.

"Relaxation 'Deskercises.'" Johns Hopkins Health Information, www.intelihealth.com, June 16, 1999.

Réquéna, Y. *Chi Kung: The Chinese Art of Mastering Energy.* Rochester, VT: Healing Arts Press, 1996.

Reuben, D. R. *Everything You Always Wanted to Know about Sex—But Were Afraid to Ask.* New York: David McKay, 1969.

Roman, M. "Your Sexual Appetite." *Men's Health*, vol. 12, issue 7, Sept. 1997, pp. 138–141.

Ryan, G. *Reclaiming Male Sexuality.* New York: M. Evans and Company, 1997.

Schwartz, K. *The Male Member.* New York: St. Martin's Press, 1985.

Scott, G. R. *Phallic Worship.* London: Luxor Press, 1966.

Sheets-Johnstone, M. *The Roots of Thinking.* Philadelphia: Temple University Press, 1990.

Shepherd, R., and S. Meyer. "Broccoli Basics." *Organic Gardening,* vol. 45, no. 2, Feb. 1998, pp. 42–44.

Simons, G. L. *The Illustrated Book of Sexual Records.* New York: Bell Publishing, 1974.

Sinatra, S. "Total Health." *Men's Health,* vol. 20, issue 4, Aug./Sept. 1998, p. 46.

Smuts, B. B., D. L. Cheney, R. M. Seyfarth, R. W. Wrangham, and T. T. Struhsaker. *Primate Societies.* Chicago: University of Chicago Press, 1987.

Strage, M. *The Durable Fig Leaf.* New York: William Morrow, 1980.

Tannahill, R. *Sex in History.* New York: Stein and Day, 1980.

Taylor, T. *The Prehistory of Sex.* New York: Bantam Books, 1996.

Vines, G. "My Best Friend's a Brussels Sprout." *New Scientist,* vol. 152, no. 2061–2, Dec. 21, 1996, pp. 46–49.

Wall, O. A. *Sex and Sex Worship.* St. Louis, MO: C. V. Mosby, 1919.

Wedeck, H. E. *A Dictionary of Aphrodisiacs.* New York: M. Evans & Co., 1992.

Wickler, W. *The Sexual Code.* Garden City, N.J.: Anchor Press, 1973.

Wincze, J. P., and M. P. Carey. *Sexual Dysfunction: A Guide for Assessment and Treatment.* New York: Guilford Press, 1991.

Wolfgan, L. A. "Charting Recent Progress: Advances in Alcohol Research." *Alcohol Health & Research World,* vol. 21, no. 4, Fall 1997, pp. 277–286.

Yesudian, S., and E. Haich. *Yoga and Health.* London: Unwin Paperbacks, 1966.

Yu, L. *The Carnal Prayer Mat.* New York: Ballantine, 1990.

Zilbergeld, B. *The New Male Sexuality.* New York: Bantam Books, 1993.

TECHNICAL BIBLIOGRAPHY

Allen, M. Individual copulatory preference and the "strange female effect" in a captive group-living male chimpanzee (pan troglodytes). *Primates,* vol. 22, 1981, pp. 221–236.

Alter, G.J. Augmentation phalloplasty. *Urologic Clinics of North America,* vol. 22, no. 4, November 1995, pp. 887–901.

Althof, S. Psychogenic impotence: Treatment of men and couples. In S. Leiblum, R. Rosen (eds.), *Principles and Practice of Sex Therapy: Update for the 1990s.* New York: Guilford, 1989.

Althof, S.E., L.A. Turner, S.B. Levine, et al. Why do so many people drop out from auto-injection therapy for impotence? *Journal of Sex and Marital Therapy,* vol. 15, no. 2, Summer 1989, pp. 121–129.

———. Intracavernosal injection in the treatment of impotence: A prospective study of sexual, psychological, and marital functioning. *Journal of Sex and Marital Therapy,* vol. 13, 1987, pp. 155–167.

———. Sexual, psychological, and marital impact of self-injection of papaverine and phentolamine: a long-term prospective study. *Journal of Sex and Marital Therapy,* vol. 17, no. 2, Summer 1991, pp. 101–112.

American Urological Association Press Release, American Urological Association panel releases treatment guideliness for impotence. Nov. 4, 1996.

Anderson, K.E., and G. Wagner. Physiology of penile erection. *Physiological Reviews,* vol. 75, no. 1, January 1995, pp. 191–236.

Bach, D., M. Schmitt, and L. Ebeling. Phytopharmaceutical and synthetic agents in the treatment of benign prostatic hyperplasia. *Phytomedicine,* vol. 3, no. 4, 1997, pp. 309–313.

Baier, D., and M. Philipp. Modification of sexual functions by antidepressants. Fortschritte der Neurologie, Psychiatrie 62, no. 1, Jan. 1994, pp. 14–21.

Ballard, S.A., L.A. Turner, and A.M. Naylor. Sildenafil, a potent selective inhibitor of type 5 phosphodiesterase, enhances nitric oxide-dependent relaxation of rabbit corpus cavernosum. *Brit J Pharmacol*, vol. 118 (Suppl.), 1996, Abst. 153P.

Balon, R. Antidepressants in the treatment of premature ejaculation. *Journal of Sex and Marital Therapy*, vol. 22, no. 2, Summer 1996, pp. 85–96.

Balon, R., V. Yeragani, R. Pohl, and C. Ramesh. Sexual dysfunction during antidepressant treatment. *J. Clin Psychiatry*, vol. 54, 1993, pp. 209–212.

Bartlik, B., P. Kaplan, and H. Kaplan. Psychostimulants apparently reverse sexual dysfunction secondary to selective serotonin re-uptake inhibitors. *Journal of Sex and Marital Therapy*, vol. 21, no. 4, Winter 1995.

Bartlik, B., P. Kaplan, and J. Kocsis. Letter to the editor: Re: Balon R: Effects of antidepressants on sexuality. *Primary Psychiatry*, vol. 2, no. 10, Nov./Dec. 1995, p. 13.

Becker, R.E. Quiz: a monthly feature. *Medical Aspects of Human Sexuality*, June 1974, pp. 169–170.

Bondil, P., P. Costa, J.P. Daures, and H. Navratil. Clinical study of the longitudinal deformation of the flaccid penis and of its variations with aging. *Eur. Urol.*, vol. 21, 1992, p. 284.

Bonnard, M. Soma and psyche: The link between the urologist and the psychiatrist in medical treatment of mixed erectile disorders. ESIR, October 4, 1997, 2nd meeting, Madrid, abstract N025, oral podium presentation.

Boolell, M., M.J. Allen, S.A. Ballard, et al. Sildenafil: an orally active type 5 cyclic GMP-specific phosphodiesterase inhibitor for the treatment of penile erectile dysfunction. *International Journal of Impotence Research*, vol. 8, no. 2, June 1996, pp. 47–52.

Boolell, M., S. Gepi-Attee, J.C. Gingell, and M.J. Allen. Sildenafil, a novel effective oral therapy for male erectile dysfunction. *Br. J. Urol.*, vol. 78, no. 2, August 1996, pp. 257–261.

Boolell, M., C. Gingell, S. Gepi-Attee, K. Wareham, and D. Price. Oral sildenafil in the treatment of penile erectile dysfunction (ED) in diabetic patients. ESIR, 2nd meeting, October 4, 1997, Madrid, abstract 7030, oral podium presentation.

Brindley, G.S. Cavernosal alpha-blockade: a new technique for investigating and treating erectile impotence. *Br J Psychiatry*, vol. 143, 1983, pp. 332–337.

Caldecoo, J.D.: Mating patterns, societies and the ecogeography of macaques. *Anim. Behav.*, vol. 34, 1986, pp. 208–220.

Cavallini, G. Minoxidil and capsaicin: an association of transcutaneous active drugs for erection facilitation (abstract). *Int J Impot Res.*, vol. 6 (suppl. 1), 1994, p. D70.

Clutton-Brock, T.H., and P.H. Harvey. Mammals, resources and reproductive strategies. *Nature*, vol. 273, 1978, pp. 181–195.

Clutton-Brock, T.H., P.H. Harvey, and B. Rudder. Sexual dimorphism, socionomic sex ratio and body weight in primates. *Nature*, vol. 269, 1977, pp. 797–800.

Cohen, A. Treatment of antidepressant-induced sexual dysfunction: a new scientific study shows benefits of ginkgo biloba. *Healthwatch*, vol. 5, no. 1, January 1996.

Dixon, A.F. Observations on the evolution of the genitalia and copulary behaviour in male primates. *J. Zool. Lond.*, vol. 213, 1987, pp. 423–443.

Donner, F., G. Wessler, R. Brown, and H. Charles. Involvement of the sympathetic nervous system in the urinary bladder internal sphincter and in penile erection in the anesthetized cat. *J Urol,* vol. 15, 1978, pp. 404–407.

Erectile dysfunction medBriefs news. *Journal of Psychosomatic Medicine,* July–August 1998.

Feldman, H.A., I. Goldstein, D.G. Hatzichristou, et al. Impotence and its medical and psychological correlates: results of the Massachusetts Male Aging Study. *J Urol,* vol. 151, January 1994, pp. 54–61.

Frank, E., C. Anderson, and D.J. Kupfer. Profiles of couples seeking sex therapy and marital therapy. *American Journal of Psychiatry,* vol. 133, 1976, pp. 559–562.

Garcia-Reboll, L., J.P. Mulhall, and I. Goldstein. Drugs for the treatment of impotence. *Drugs and Aging,* vol. 11, no. 2, August 1997, pp. 140–151.

Giuliano, F., Rampin O., and A. Jardin. Physiology of erection. *Rev Med Intern,* vol. 18 (suppl. 1), 1997, pp. 3S-9S.

Goldstein, I., T.F. Lue, H. Padma-Nathan, et al. Oral sildenafil in the treatment of erectile dysfunction. *N Eng J Med,* vol. 338, no. 20, May 14, 1998, pp. 1397–1404.

Ito, T., K. Kawahara, A. Das, and W. Strudwick. The effects of ArginMax, a natural dietary supplement for enhancement of male sexual function. *Hawaii Medical Journal,* vol. 57, no. 12, December 1998, p. 741.

Jamison, P.L., and P.H. Gebhard. Penis size increase between flaccid and erect state: An analysis of the Kinsey data. *J. Sex Res.,* vol. 24, 1988, p. 177.

Jeremy, J.Y., S.A. Ballard, A.M. Naylor, et al. The effects of sildenafil, an inhibitor of type 5 cGMP phosphodiesterase, on cGMP and cAMP levels in rabbit corpus cavernosum, in vitro. *Brit J Pharmacol,* vol. 119 (suppl.), 1996, Abst 84P.

Kaiser, F.E., and S.G. Korenman. Impotence in diabetic men. *American Journal of Medicine,* suppl. 5A, 1988, pp. 147–152.

Kaplan, H.S. The combined use of sex therapy and intrapenile injections in the treatment of impotence. *Journal of Sex and Marital Therapy,* vol. 16, 1990, p. 195.

Kegel, A. Sexual functions of the pubo-coccygeus muscle. *W.J. Surg. Obst. Gyn.,* vol. 60, 1952, p. 521.

Kelton, P.L. Principles of skin grafts. *Selected Readings in Plastic Surgery,* vol. 6, 1990, no. 2.

Kim, N., K.M. Azadzoi, I. Goldstein, and I. Saenz de Tejada. A nitric oxide-like factor mediates on-adrenergic-noncholinergic neurogenic relaxation of penile corpus cavernosum smooth muscle. *J. Clin Invest,* vol. 88, 1991, pp. 112–118.

Korenman, S.G. New insights into erectile dysfunction: a practical approach. *American Journal of Medicine,* vol. 105, issue 2, August 1998, p. 135.

Krane, R.J., I. Goldstein, and I. Saenz de Tejada. Medical progress on impotence. *New England Journal of Medicine,* vol. 321, no. 24, Dec. 14, 1989, pp. 1648–1659.

Krauss, D.J., L.J. Lantinga, and C.M. Kelly. In treating impotence, urology and sex therapy are complementary. *Urology,* vol. 36, no. 5, November 1990, pp. 467–470.

Levine, L.A., and E.L. Lenting. Use of nocturnal penile tumescence and rigidity in the evaluation of male erectile dysfunction. *Urol. Clin. North Am.,* vol. 22, 1995, pp. 775–788.

McCulloch, D.K., I.W. Campbell, F.C. Wu, et al. The prevalence of diabetic impotence. *Diabetologia,* vol. 18, 1980, pp. 279–283.

Mitka, M. Viagra leads as rivals are moving up. *The Journal of the American Medical Association,* vol. 280, no. 2, July 8, 1998, p.119.

Montague, D.K., J.H. Barada, A.M. Belker, et al. Clinical guidelines panel on erectile dysfunction: summary report on the treatment of organic erectile dysfunction. *Journal of Urology*, vol. 156, December 1996, pp. 2007–2011.

Morales, A., M. Condra, J. Owen, et al. Is yohimbine effective in the treatment of organic impotence? Results of a controlled trial. *Journal of Urology*, vol. 137, 1987, p. 1168.

Morales, A., M. Condra, and K. Reid. The role of nocturnal penile tumescence monitoring in the diagnosis of impotence, a review. *Journal of Urology*, vol. 143, 1990, pp. 441–446.

Morales, A., J.P. Heaton, B. Johnston, and M. Adams. Oral and topical treatment of erectile dysfunction: Present and future. *Urol Clin North Am*, vol. 22, no. 4, November 1995, pp. 879–886.

Morley, J.E., and F.E. Kaiser. Impotence in elderly men. *Drugs and Aging*, vol. 2, no. 4, 1992, pp. 330–344.

Mulhall, J. Sildenafil: a novel effective oral therapy for male erectile dysfunction. *British Journal of Urology*, vol. 79, 1997, pp. 661–664.

NIH Consensus Statement. "Impotence." December 7–9 1992. Vol. 10, no. 4, 1992, pp. 1–31.

Prescott, E., et al. Alcohol intake and the risk of lung cancer. *American Journal of Epidemiology*, vol. 149, March 1, 1999, pp. 463–470.

Riley, A.J. Yohimbine in the treatment of erectile disorder. *The British Journal of Clinical Practice*, vol. 48, no. 3, May/June 1994, pp. 133–36.

Rimm, E.B., M.J. Stampfer, A. Ascherio, et al. Vitamin E consumption and the risk of coronary heart disease in men. *New England Journal of Medicine*, vol. 328, 1993, pp. 1450–56.

Rothschild, A.J. Selective serotonin reuptake inhibitor-induced sexual dysfunction: efficacy of a drug holiday. *Am J. Psychiatry,* vol. 152, 1995, pp. 1514–1516.

Thase, M.E, C.F. Reynolds, L.M. Glans, et al. Nocturnal penile tumescence in depressed men. *Am J. Psychiatry,* vol. 144, 1987, pp. 89–92.

Tiefer, L., and D. Schuetz-Mueller. Psychological issues in diagnosis and treatment of erectile disorders. Urologic Clinics of North America, vol. 22, no. 4, November 1995, pp. 767–774.

Verinis, J.S., and S. Roll. Primary and secondary male characteristics: the hairiness and large penis stereotypes. *Psychological Reports,* vol. 26, 1970, pp. 123–126.

Wessels, H., T.F. Lue, and J.W. McNinch. Penile length in the flaccid and erect states: guidelines for penile augmentation. *Journal of Urology,* vol. 156, September 1996, pp. 995–997.

Wise, T.N. Sexual dysfunction in the medically ill. *Psychosomatics,* vol. 24, 1983, pp. 787–801.

Zorgniotti, A., and R. Lefleur. Auto-injection of the corpus cavernosum with a vasoactive drug combination for vasculogenic impotence. *Journal of Urology,* vol. 133, 1985, pp. 39–41.

RESOURCES

American Association of Sex Educators,
Counselors and Therapists
P.O. Box 238
Mount Vernon, IA 52314-0238

American Diabetes Association
National Center
1660 Duke Street
Alexandria, VA 22314
800-232-3472
Website: http://www.diabetes.org

American Foundation for Urological Disease
1128 North Charles Street
Baltimore, MD 21201
800-242-2383 or 410-468-1800
Website: http://www.afud.org

Caverject
Pharmaceutical Informational Associates Ltd.
2761 Trenton Road
Levittown, PA 19056
800-867-7042 or 215-949-0490

Website: http://www.pharminfo.com/pubs/msb/
caverject.html
Also: www.impotent.com/whatis.html

Glenwood and Western Medical
82 North Summit Street
Tenafly, NJ 07670
800-237-9083
Website: http://www.glenwood-llc.com

Herb Research Foundation
1007 Pearl Street
Suite 200
Boulder, CO 80302
800-748-2617 or 303-449-2265
Fax: 303-449-7849
Website: http://www.herbs.org

Impotence Anonymous
119 South Ruth Street
Maryville, TN 37801-5746

Impotence Hotline
800-433-4215

Impotence Information Center
P.O. Box 9, Dept. USA
Minneapolis, MN 55440
800-543-9632

Impotence Institute of America
P.O. Box 410
Bowie, MD 20718-0410
800-669-1603
Website: http://www.impotenceworld.org

Johan's Guide to Aphrodisiacs
Website: http://www.207.158.197.112/
aphrodisaphrhome.htm

Men's Consultation Clinic
at Johns Hopkins Hospital
410-955-6707

Netrition
20 Petra Lane
Albany, NY 12205
888-817-2411
Fax: 518-456-9673
Website: http://www.netrition.com

Not For Men Only
The Male Health Center
400 West LBJ Freeway
Suite 360
Irving, TX 75063
972-751-6253
Website: http://www.malehealthcenter.com

Pfizer's
U.S. Pharmaceuticals
888-484-2472
Website: http://www.viagra.com

Raintree Nutrition, Inc.
1601 W. Koenig Lane
Austin, TX 78756
800- 780-5902 or 512-467-6130
Fax: 512-467-6822
Website: http://www.rain-tree.com

Sex Information & Education Council of U.S.
130 West 42nd Street
New York, NY 10036
212-819-9770

Timm Medical Systems
6541 City West Parkway
Eden Prairie, MN 55344
800-344-9688 or 800-438-8592
Website: http://www.timmmedical.com
Also: www.erectionsolution.com

Vet-Co, Inc.
3700 5th Avenue South
Birmingham, AL 35222
800-827-8382
Fax: 205-595-3845
Website: http://www.vetcoinc.com
Also: www.jax-ads.com/impotence/vetco.htm

Vivus, Inc.
605 East Fairchild Drive
Mountain View, CA 94043
888-367-6873
Website: http://www.vivus.com

Women's Sexual Health Clinic
at Boston University
617-638-8555

INDEX